PSYCHOTHERAPY, ANTHROPOLOGY AND THE WORK OF CULTURE

Anthropology and psychotherapy have a long and important historical relationship, and in this fascinating collection practitioners with experience in both fields explore how the concept of 'culture' is deployed to guide and frame contemporary therapeutic theory, training and practice.

This task is particularly important as the global spread of psychotherapy, as both an outgrowth of and a potential point of critique to globalised hyper-capitalism, requires us to think differently about how to conceptualise cultural difference in psychotherapy.

Psychotherapy, Anthropology and the Work of Culture provides a valuable resource for psychotherapeutic professionals working in a world in which cultural difference appears in fluid and transient moments. It will also provide essential reading for students and researchers working across the fields of psychotherapy and anthropology.

Keir Martin is Associate Professor of Social Anthropology at the University of Oslo and was previously Lecturer in Social Anthropology at the University of Manchester. He has conducted ethnographic fieldwork in East New Britain Province, Papua New Guinea, and is a member of the British Association for Counselling and Psychotherapy.

PSYCHOTHERAPY, ANTHROPOLOGY AND THE WORK OF CULTURE

Edited by Keir Martin

Routledge
Taylor & Francis Group
LONDON AND NEW YORK

First published 2019
by Routledge
2 Park Square, Milton Park, Abingdon, Oxon OX14 4RN

and by Routledge
52 Vanderbilt Avenue, New York, NY 10017

Routledge is an imprint of the Taylor & Francis Group, an informa business

British Library Cataloguing-in-Publication Data
A catalogue record for this book is available from the British Library

Library of Congress Cataloging-in-Publication Data
A catalog record for this book has been requested

ISBN: 978-0-367-18245-8 (hbk)
ISBN: 978-0-367-18251-9 (pbk)
ISBN: 978-0-429-06031-1 (ebk)

Typeset in Bembo
by Apex CoVantage, LLC

CONTENTS

AUTHOR BIOGRAPHIES

Vincent Crapanzano is Distinguished Professor of Anthropology and Comparative Literature at the Graduate Center of the City University of New York (CUNY). He has written extensively on psychoanalysis and its application to the human sciences. His latest book is *Recapitulations: A Memoir.*

James Davies graduated from the University of Oxford in 2006 with a PhD in Social and Medical Anthropology. He is a Reader in Social Anthropology and Psychotherapy at the University of Roehampton and a practicing psychotherapist. He has delivered lectures at Harvard, Yale, Oxford, Brown, UCL and Columbia and has written for *The Times*, the *New Scientist*, the *Guardian* and *Salon*. He is author of the bestselling book *Cracked: Why Psychiatry Is Doing More Harm Than Good* (Icon), and *The Making of Psychotherapists* (Karnac). He is Co-Founder of the Council for Evidence-Based Psychiatry.

Sudhir Kakar is a psychoanalyst and writer. He has been a lecturer at Harvard University, Visiting Professor at the Universities of Chicago, McGill, Melbourne, Hawaii, Vienna, and INSEAD, and Fellow at the Institutes of Advanced Study, Princeton and Berlin. Kakar is the author of fourteen books of non-fiction and six novels.

Junko Kitanaka, PhD, is a professor of anthropology in the Department of Human Sciences at Keio University, Tokyo. She was born and educated in Japan before obtaining an MA at the University of Chicago and a PhD at McGill University under Margaret Lock and Allan Young. She has been conducting research on psychiatry for two decades, collaborating globally with doctors and anthropologists, teaching in Japan and advising graduate students from the U.S. and Europe, while helping organize international conferences including the

2015 World Congress of Asian Psychiatry. She has received a number of awards, including the 2007 Dissertation Award from the American Anthropological Association's Society for Medical Anthropology. Her dissertation has since been published by Princeton University Press as a 2012 book titled *Depression in Japan: Psychiatric Cures for a Society in Distress*, which won the American Anthropological Association's Francis Hsu Prize for Best Book in East Asian Anthropology in 2013. The book has been translated by Dr Pierre-Henri Castel at the University of Paris-Descartes and published by D'Ithaque as *De la mort voluntaire au suicide au travail: Histoire et anthropologie de la depression au Japon* (2014). She is currently working on a new project on health screening and preventive medicine in the workplace; psychotherapy and trauma care in the post-nuclear age; and the medicalization of the lifecycle (developmental disorders, depression and dementia). Junko has served on the editorial boards of *Biosocieties, Medical Anthropology Quarterly and Cultural Anthropology.* Her recent publications include: The Rebirth of Secrets and the New Care of the Self in Depressed Japan. *Current Anthropology* 56(12): S251–S262, 2015; *Depression as a Problem of Labor: Japanese Debates About Work, Stress, and a New Therapeutic Ethos*; and *Sadness or Depression?: International Perspectives on the Depression Epidemic and Its Meaning*, Jerome Wakefield & Steeves Demazeux eds. Springer, 2016.

Inga-Britt Krause was trained as a social anthropologist and now works as Consultant Systemic Psychotherapist in the Tavistock & Portman NHS Foundation Trust, where she is also Training & Development Consultant and Lead for the Systemic Psychotherapy Professional Doctorate programme. Her work has focused on anti-discrimination in mental health service and psychotherapy delivery in the National Health Service in the UK and on 'culture' as a territory for resistance and denial in psychotherapy theory and practice.

Tanya Luhrmann is the Watkins University Professor at Stanford University, in the Stanford Anthropology Department. Her work focuses on the edge of experience: on voices, visions, the world of the supernatural and the world of psychosis. She has done ethnography on the streets of Chicago with homeless and psychotic women and worked with people who hear voices in Chennai, Accra and the South Bay. She has also done fieldwork with evangelical Christians who seek to hear God speak back; with Zoroastrians who set out to create a more mystical faith; and with people who practice magic. She uses a combination of ethnographic and experimental methods to understand the phenomenology of unusual sensory experiences, the way they are shaped by ideas about minds and persons, and what we can learn from this social shaping that can help us to help those whose voices are distressing. She was elected to the American Academy of Arts and Sciences in 2003 and received a John Guggenheim Fellowship award in 2007. *When God Talks Back* was named a NYT Notable Book of the Year and a Kirkus Reviews Best Book of the Year. It was awarded the $100,000 Grawemeyer Prize for Religion by the University of Louisville. She has published over thirty OpEds in the *New York Times*, and her work has been featured in the *New Yorker*, the *New York Review of Books*, the *Times Literary Supplement*, *Science News* and many other publications. Her new book, *Our Most Troubling Madness: Schizophrenia and Culture*, was published by the University of California Press in October 2016.

Keir Martin, PhD, is Associate Professor of Social Anthropology at the University of Oslo. He obtained a PhD in Anthropology at the University of Manchester and later qualified as a psychotherapist. His main areas of research have been in the field of the relationship between contested subjectivities and emerging forms of social stratification. He previously worked as a volunteer therapist at a prison in Greater Manchester. He is currently organising a research project to look at the spread of psychotherapy in the emerging 'BRIC' economies and works in private psychotherapy practice in Oslo.

Karen Seeley is Lecturer in Anthropology at Columbia University and teaches in the Psychology Department at Barnard College. She is the author of *Cultural Psychotherapy: Working With Culture in the Clinical Encounter* (2000) and *Therapy After Terror: 9/11, Psychotherapists and Mental Health* (2008). She has a private psychotherapy practice, working with individuals and couples and specializing in intercultural treatment.

Salma Siddique, PhD, is Director for Counselling and Psychotherapy in the School of Education at the University of Aberdeen, Scotland. She obtained her doctorate in anthropology from the University of St. Andrews and later qualified as a psychotherapist and clinical supervisor. Her main research interests are based on the dialogue between psychoanalysis, psychotherapy and anthropology and are influenced by her clinical experience working with people in trauma resulting from torture and fleeing conflict zones. Salma continues to practice as a volunteer psychotherapist. She supervises trainees and qualified psychotherapists and counsellors in their practices.

PREFACE

The time has come for anthropologists and psychotherapists to pay serious attention to each other. This may not seem obvious. The resonances between the two endeavors is evident to those who know both, but to those who do not, the idea that they should learn from each other might seem not only confused but even repugnant. The critical, assumption-challenging stance of anthropology can seem threatening to psychotherapists seeking to assert empirical validity to medical science. The focus on the psychological can seem wrong-headed to anthropologists focused on power and social structure.

Yet what therapists and ethnographers do is remarkably alike. Both involve participant observation. At least, ethnography straightforwardly involves the attempt to participate, to the extent possible, as a member of the group the ethnographer has come to study, and the attempt to observe what one must do in order to be recognized as a member of that group. On the surface, psychotherapy does not seem like that at all – except that in practice it is so similar that Harry Stack Sullivan actually called it "participant observation." His premise was that the psychotherapist is not the Freudian blank screen, on which the patient projects his fantasies. Instead, the psychotherapist is better understood as a person who enters into the life world of the patient as an interlocutor, with the goal of observing it closely enough that they can describe what they learn about the life-world's implicit rules and expectations. Meanwhile, the skills of ethnographic observation bear some resemblance to the skills of clinical observation and to some extent are taught in a similar manner, through apprenticeship and supervision. The ethnographer listens and tries to understand, rather than to judge; the ethnographer returns to the subject to try to corroborate the ethnographic insights (an insight being not unlike an interpretation); and the ethnographer works with the subject to develop a sense of how the subject sees and experiences their world.

Moreover, both psychotherapists and ethnographers understand more deeply than most people that the accounts they give of what they observe – their insights and interpretations – are partial and co-constructed. Insights and interpretations are, to some extent at least, narrative truths rather than historical truths. People are complicated, and any attempt to capture a person's motivations and experiences is flawed.

The difference between psychotherapy and ethnography, of course, is that the therapist is trying to change the other person through participant-observation, and the anthropologist is not. The therapist is using participant-observation to help the person with whom they work to understand themselves so that they can change. Anthropologists often imagine themselves as trying to alter the world they study as little as possible and to describe it as carefully as they can in order to make some point in an intellectual argument their research subjects will never read.

This is why the two fields can learn from each other.

These days, anthropologists have a harder and harder time seeing the point of their own arguments. We are at an unusually morose moment in our discipline's history. No grand debates captivate the field. Our theoretical lodestones have not changed much since the 1970s, when we fell in love with Foucault and power became an explanatory axis. Our research topics have grown far more diverse that they were for our intellectual ancestors, but the world itself has become less varied – more accessible, more interconnected, more travelled. No one will ever be able to write a book like *Witchcraft, Oracles and Magic Among the Azande* and startle an Oxford senior common room in the same way again.

What anthropology can learn from psychotherapy is that their work matters when it has the potential to change the lives of those among whom we work. If we thought of the audience for our work as including those among whom we work, our field would change. Our work would become more readable, for a start. We would also be forced to ask whether what we learned in our research was worth the investment of our participant's time: whether what we learned about the symptoms of depression in some particular place, for example, was relevant to thinking about the treatment of depression, so that clinicians treating depression there might learn something useful. This does not mean that anthropology should become applied. It is more that when one does research on questions to which one's research subjects want to know the answers, the work seems more meaningful and more alive. Students who asked questions like these would find a greater sense of purpose.

What psychotherapists can learn from anthropology is that culture is not something you possess but something you do (to use James Davies' formulation here). The great pressure on the practice of psychotherapy within a socially diverse world is to show that people from different backgrounds can benefit from this care. Thus, a new emphasis on "cultural competence" has emerged. But it is all too easy to allow an attention to cultural difference to become a parade of stereotypes. Anthropologists know that culture is what participant observation discovers through the interaction between people. The central principle in cultural competence should be respect in the interaction with other people – not knowledge about who one thinks those other people are.

The greatest stakes, however, are that anthropologists and psychotherapists can build together an awareness-centered model of the mind. This is what I see at the heart of Keir Martin's project here. There are many scientists working to develop accounts of mental process from what Heinz Kohut, and later Clifford Geertz, called an experience-distant perspective – and we need those accounts. But we also need accounts that pay close attention to the experience of thinking, believing, desiring, imagining, feeling, and so forth. Anthropologists and psychotherapists have more experience-near knowledge about the way people experience mental states than scholars and practitioners in any other fields. Working across fields, they will be able to ask whether the subtle accounts of human experience people learn from depth exploration in a clinical context make sense in a non-clinical context in another culture, and how the knowledge of those non-clinical domains should challenge the assumptions within the consulting room. From these exchanges – and particularly from those who are both ethnographically and clinically sophisticated – will come a more complete understanding of the mind that we have had, and of the self, the person, the imagination, and of social life in general.

Tanja Luhrmann

ACKNOWLEDGEMENTS

This book came out of a series of workshops hosted and supported by the Department of Social Anthropology at the University of Oslo. I would like to thank the Department for their support in making this book possible. I would also like to thank all of the participants in the workshops and the writing project for their input. In particular, I would like to mention Kate Schechter of Chicago University. Although Kate was unable to contribute a written piece to this volume, her contribution to the discussions was an important part of the process that led to this book. In addition, I would like to thank a series of interlocuters from the Manchester Psychotherapy community for discussions, in particular Karen Burke, Fatima Adam, Sue Hawkins, Andrew Hodges, Tayeba Jaleel, Angela Keane and Tom Keeley. I would also like to thank my co-collaborators in establishing the European Network for Psychological Anthropology, James Davies and Thomas Stodulka. And, finally, I would like to thank the staff at Karnac Books and Routledge for their help and encouragement in this process.

INTRODUCTION

Keir Martin

Psychotherapy stands accused. The charge sheet consists of old familiar indictments made from new and surprising quarters. At the top of the list is the claim that psychotherapy embodies an individualism that it is both unable and unwilling to fully explore. The cure is classically psychodynamic. It consists of bringing to awareness and working through the unconscious origin of this now taken for granted way of being in the world. Hence, the foundation of psychotherapy's character is both the hidden cause and the potentially to-be-revealed cure of its currently diagnosed pathology. Psychotherapy's 'individualism' is caused by its origins in a particular cultural setting. For those who speak in general terms, this is 'the West'. For those with more of an interest in the particular case of Freudian psychoanalysis, it is the narrower context of 1890s middle-class Vienna. Either way, because of its cultural origin, psychotherapy has allegedly focused on the internal lives of bounded individuals, and because of this singular focus, it is said to have remained blind to the importance of culture. Like a client trapped by maladaptive ways of seeing, feeling and being that originate from her upbringing in a dysfunctional family that her current dysfunction leaves her unable to perceive and break, so psychotherapy itself is characterised as being trapped within a similar tragic unconscious feedback loop with regard to the culture that brought it into being. The increasingly widely accepted remedy is to bring this dysfunctional model to awareness so that its negative effects and absences can be recognised and new, healthier ways of seeing put in its place. Psychotherapy is enjoined to bring culture to its own therapeutic awareness. In this telling of the story, then, the cure for psychotherapy's culturally determined malaise is revealed to be the revelation of culture.

These are in some regards not new complaints. They are almost as old as psychoanalysis and modern psychotherapy, and they will be familiar to anyone with an interest in the more critical edges of psychotherapeutic theory or social scientific discussions of the limitations of Western psychotherapy. The critique of psychotherapy's alleged focus on the bounded individual and its concomitant ignorance of culture is perhaps most associated with the discipline of anthropology, where it has a long history dating back at least as far as Malinowski's debates with Ernest Jones in the 1920s regarding the universality of the Oedipus complex. These discussions set the template for a recurring discussion inside anthropology that pitted universalist explanations of human existence (such as those allegedly given by classical psychoanalysis) against cultural relativist critiques of the alleged ethnocentric assumptions of such models. In recent years, such criticisms have gained a new audience and importance, however. No longer the preserve of critics on or outside the borders of the therapeutic community, they have been incorporated into the heart of psychotherapeutic theory, training and practice. Although some may continue to decry mention of cultural difference as heresy or a defence mechanism against the universal truths discovered by their particular school of thought, 'culture' is now an essential component of many therapy training courses, taking up as much, or more, space and time than concepts such as 'transference' or 'empathy'. And even if in some quarters the nature of its introduction is resisted, isn't such resistance to the revelation of blind spots in the patient's way of seeing herself an inevitable part of the process of change? Great effort goes into overcoming this resistance to 'culture', just as previous generations of analysts might have put great effort into identifying clients' references to their 'culture' as a defence mechanism designed to resist the revelation of a hidden truth. 'Cultural' competence has gone from being an invisible or unmentioned factor to a core competence that must be seen to be acknowledged and performed.

This recent and sudden incorporation of 'culture' into the heart of contemporary psychotherapy coincides with other changes. Most notable are moves towards the manualisation and standardisation of psychotherapy training and provision. With this has come a greater emphasis on the demonstration of acquiring particular skills and competences to deal with particular issues, as opposed to a perspective that viewed the acquisition of such skills more as a means to the development of a particular holistic, therapeutically beneficial subjectivity or way of being. That the rise to prominence of a particular model of demonstrating 'cultural competence' should coincide with these other changes of emphasis and governance may not be entirely coincidental, as many of the contributors to this volume argue.

THE CRITIQUE OF THERAPEUTIC 'INDIVIDUALISM'

Let us start with the 'individualism' of which therapy is now accused and the problems that it is said to carry with it. 'Individualism', we are told is 'Western'. Consequently, any explicit claim or implicit underlying assumption that such 'individualism' is the starting point for understanding persons or the desired end point of therapeutic intervention is said to be potentially illustrative of an arrogant and ethnocentric attitude. In recent years, this critique has gone from being predominantly an academic or political critique made from the outside to one that is increasingly internally enforced as a new orthodoxy to which practitioners must themselves display affiliation. This process has taken on a new urgency within the discipline as psychotherapy spreads globally and as its client base in its Western heartlands becomes more 'culturally' diverse. Performing this new acquired understanding can then be added to the set of core competencies that 'best practice' or the 'professionalization' of psychotherapy requires in an increasingly standardised, regulated and institutionally managed age.

A defining characteristic of the 'individualism', allegedly so central to the kind of psychotherapy critiqued in these depictions, is an obsessive focus on the interior of the person at the expense of the external social relations and structures within which they are embedded. Far from 'individualism' being a 'natural' state at constant risk of being crushed by an over-regulating society, as in some libertarian perspectives, 'individualism' from this perspective can itself become conceptualised as an ideology or way of being imposed by a competitive society upon persons who may otherwise have gravitated towards more communal or consensual ways of being. It is worth noting that there has long been a strand of criticism of psychotherapy that has contrasted its alleged obsessive individualism with its reciprocal ignorance of external factors, particularly from those on the political left, both within and outside the discipline that has tried to question the extent to which psychotherapy necessarily adapts its clients to the needs of a competitive society or might instead be part of a radical critique of that society's foundational premises.

Today perspectives that are critical of therapeutic 'individualism' are more likely to conceptualise such external networks of relations and ideas as 'culture' than 'society', and along with that shift has come other shifts of emphasis. The rise of 'culture' as the concept to be contrasted to the 'individual' in such discussions coincides with a downgrading of the importance of 'economic' factors that itself goes alongside a growing tendency to frame the problem to be addressed as one of cultural misrecognition of non-individualist ways of being. This in turn coincides with a situation where it is broadly agreed that working and wage-labour are good practices in which people should be encouraged to participate. Work is often framed as a social good, and therapy's funding by governments and business interests has often depended upon demonstrating that it can help to achieve that social good. Recent expansions of business and government support for therapy, such as were seen in the UK in the early 2000s, were explicitly linked to this perceived social good, and expanded therapy services, such as IAPT, were set the explicit task of getting more people back to work. This coincides with a situation where statistical evidence is marshalled to support the idea that getting back to work is good for depressed or emotionally unwell patients and predicts a better chance of 'recovery'. The possibility that the entire structure of work in contemporary society might create illness and dissatisfaction both for those who are able to secure and hold employment and those who are not was largely removed from the agenda. *This* particular wider social criticism, which one can easily imagine being put forward by previous psychotherapeutic radicals such as Fromm, Laing or David Cooper, no longer fits a zeitgeist in which the acceptance of the healthiness of work is a precondition for funding and support.

INDIVIDUALISM AND THE INNER PERSON

The Western individualism allegedly at the heart of psychotherapy stands accused of an excessive focus on the interior of the individual. It is a focus that is often described as misunderstanding the nature of human beings in general as being the outcome of some innate inner essence contained within the individual as a bounded entity. If the problem is determined to be 'individualist' or 'psychological' therapy's lack of (attention to) the wider 'culture', then the addition of 'culture' to therapy almost inexorably presents itself as the obvious solution to therapy's shortcomings. The chapters in this collection critically engage with some of the issues raised by the move towards this framing from a variety of angles. All of the contributors to this volume are professional anthropologists or ethnographers, and all but two are fully qualified psychoanalysts or psychotherapists, with the remaining two both having made research on psychotherapy and psychoanalysis a central aspect of their anthropological work. Anthropology and psychotherapy have had an at times long and fruitful relationship, but it is a relationship that has often been dogged by mutual antagonism and misunderstanding. The role of 'individualism' in classical psychotherapy is possibly one of those misunderstandings, and it is arguably a misunderstanding that is now being imported back wholesale into contemporary psychotherapy from external sources such as anthropology. The concept of 'culture' that is becoming increasingly important within psychotherapy is one that was largely developed within anthropology, although that discipline has now largely discarded the particular conceptualisation of 'culture' that contemporary psychotherapy increasingly makes use of. These are issues that those with a foot in both camps are in a unique position to explore, and through a variety of contemporary and historical analyses they aim to shed light on some historical and current expressions of this ongoing relationship.

In the remainder of this introduction, I explore some of what anthropology and psychotherapy may illuminate in each other today. In particular, I explore some of the background to the current suspicion of 'individualism' and the attempt to correct its shortcomings with the addition of 'culture'. This is an issue with a long pedigree. If anything, it is *the* issue that has defined the long and sometimes problematic relationship between anthropology and psychotherapy. Rather than revisit a history that has been told elsewhere, one of the aims of this collection is to explore the terms of the debate as it is currently being conducted in psychotherapy in the midst of its 'cultural' turn. Anthropological theory has devoted much effort in the past few decades to encouraging a greater attention to the shifting meaning of words and concepts (including 'culture') and how these words and concepts shape those contexts as much as they describe them. Rather than assuming that 'culture' or 'individualism' are concepts which simply refer to clearly defined aspects of human existence, the focus is increasingly on the work that these concepts do to create a separation between aspects of existence and thereby reshape that existence. The implication of this as a starting point might be to carry a degree of scepticism towards the assumption that psychotherapy simply expresses something called 'Western individualism', and to instead begin our discussions by considering what is meant by 'individualism' in any particular context, such as the therapy room or therapy training classroom, and to try to explore what the speaker wishes to achieve by deploying and framing the concept in that particular way.

BEYOND THE 'BOUNDED' INDIVIDUAL

The 'individualism' that many contemporary critiques of psychotherapy seek to deconstruct is one that is said to construct individual persons as if they were bounded autonomous entities (see Martin this volume). In this conception, individuals may enter into relations with others, but the nature of those relations is fundamentally determined by an innate essence contained within the bounds of this individual human entity. The implication of this is that the individual self becomes both the starting point of theory and the end point of practical interventions designed to improve the human condition, rather than the networks of social relations within which persons are entangled and formed (see also Siddique this volume).

Different versions of this conception are indeed common in the history of Western thought, as contemporary critics of individual 'psychological' therapy such as John McLeod observe. It can be identified as the basis of many of the foundational texts of Western political theory, such as Hobbes and Locke, who despite their manifold differences arguably have variants of this conception of human being at the heart of their intellectual projects (e.g. Macpherson 1962). Likewise, mainstream neoclassical economic theory can be described as being largely built upon this framework, while Freud is often read, by supporters and opponents alike, as also standing in this tradition. His theory of innate drives that shape social relations can all too easily be read as a sexualised version of the aggressive urges or economic propensities that Hobbes and Locke respectively saw as providing the need for a society or state that regulates those destructive tendencies.

While this conception of human being has been massively influential in 'the West' over the past five centuries, so too have been other formations that have often explicitly challenged this foundation. Early twentieth-century anthropology advanced one such challenge, with its attempt to demonstrate the particular 'Western' nature of this conception of human being through a contrast with less 'individualistic' conceptions that were allegedly more prominent among non-Western peoples. From the second half of the twentieth century, this ethnographic work was increasingly taken up by sociologists and anthropologists working in more 'Western' environments. This work has frequently demonstrated the ways in which 'Western' persons often have a far more ambivalent relationship to 'individualism' and a far more 'relational' conception of their own nature than a simple 'West as individualism' paradigm might allow for. There is a long history in Western social thought of visions that challenge or nuance bounded individualism, of which the classical anthropological 'cultural relativist' critique that is now being introjected wholesale into psychotherapy is merely one example.

This point is important to make, as on occasion the nature of what is meant by 'individualism' can be taken for granted along with its association with the 'West'. One can all too easily end up assuming that there is simple global separation between the 'West' as a culture, where a particular kind of individualism rules supreme, and the 'rest', where it does not. In fact, the Western world is full of debate and discussion about 'individualism' and an often-pained exploration of the ambiguities arising from it. How many politicians have praised individual initiative as the basis of an entrepreneurial society one day, for example, and then denounced rising 'individualism' as a threat to social order the next? Rather than being portrayed as a world-view that expresses a fixed underlying Western individualism, psychotherapy might instead be seen as one of the key locations in twentieth-century thought for an exploration of the ambiguities of individualism. Instead of simply seeing psychotherapy as in need of socio-cultural input from anthropology, a more nuanced understanding of psychotherapy's history might lead us to see the ways in which psychotherapy has long been dealing with many of the self-same issues concerning the relational construction of persons with which contemporary anthropology finds itself battling, as it attempts to move beyond older perspectives premised on diagnosing the nature of the relationship between the 'individual' and her 'society' or 'culture'.

In their different ways, most psychotherapeutic theories have explicitly or implicitly destabilised the very nature of the distinction between the inside and the outside of the person that is the assumed starting point for contemporary critics, such as McLeod's vision both of the drawbacks of (internally focused) 'psychological' therapy and for the (externally focused) 'cultural' therapy that will correct its shortcomings. McLeod describes a series of foci for traditional psychological therapies, as if they simply demonstrate a focus on the interior of the bounded individual that unites all the different therapeutic schools. This even includes modalities, such as Object Relations, that explicitly focus on relations as the foundation of the development of the person. Object Relations' focus on the interplay of social relations across the boundary of the self might lead one to conclude that its vision of the person is in many regards diametrically opposed to that of a bounded entity whose existence precedes relations. Indeed, its focus on the *interiorisation* of relations suggests that the very core of the person is relational and that *it is the process of creating a distinction between relations that are internalised and those that are left external that makes a person.* Far from a distinction between an outside world of culture and relations and an inner world of essence being the inevitable starting point in which we have to pick one side or another, Kleinian therapy and its inheritors in the British Independent School might suggest a starting point in which relations themselves are primary, both *inside and outside.* This does not mean that the distinction between inside and outside might not be important, but it is a distinction that cannot be assumed and has rather to be forged in practice. One potential course would be to further theoretically explore the ways in which Object Relations destabilises the very idea of a fixed boundary between inside and outside. Instead, the contemporary 'cultural' critique takes Object Relations' focus on the interiorisation of particular relations (a process that actually creates the very nature of an 'interior') as evidence that Object Relations can safely be packaged alongside all the other 'Western' therapies as having a focus on bounded autonomous individual subjects. So, McLeod (2002:137) informs us that new 'cultural' forms of therapy focus on therapy as a, 'discursive arena'.

> The idea of therapy as a discursive arena is, of course, quite contrary to most existing understandings of therapy, which postulate some kind of inner mechanism or structure within the individual (self, object relations, cognitive or emotional schema) that is deficient and requires restoration.

We could note that the idea of therapy as a 'discursive arena' may not seem so alien to many 'existing understandings of therapy' as McLeod seems to suggest, going as far back as Freud and Breur's popularisation of Anna O's term, 'the talking cure', in the late nineteenth century. More important, in McLeod's depiction, Object Relations (as conceived by Kleinians or British Independents or (presumably) contemporary US relational psychoanalysts) are simply cast as internal, while 'discursive arena[s]' are simply cast as external. But can such phenomena be divided and packaged up in this manner? After all, 'internal dialogue' is one of the most fundamental processes of human existence and reflection. Like (object) relations, language is a fundamentally social phenomenon. Language is an intersubjective social phenomenon that exists both within and without the individual person simultaneously in a manner that often makes her boundaries appear anything but clear and bounded. In McLeod's characterisation of Object Relations, he takes two phenomena – (object) relations and language – that are both intrinsically social and show the intrinsically social nature of even the core of the person, and show how they exist both within and without the person. He then takes one (Object Relations, whose very necessity for 'internalisation' suggests a foundational position beyond inside/outside) and places it on the inside, and another (language) and places it on the outside, in order to preserve a distinction between psychological and cultural therapies in which the former can all be jointly condemned for their 'individualism'. Here, he reproduces a debate that has a long provenance in anthropological theory over the manner and extent to which it is always possible to sharply distinguish between inner and outer states of being. This distinction was fundamental to much traditional anthropological analysis, and it is this focus on the 'external' factors of society or culture as the proper focus for anthropological endeavour that explains much of the disdain for 'psychologising' that has often characterised the discipline, as Davies (this volume) observes. Hence, to take one example, the influential post-war British anthropologist, Sir Edmund Leach (1958:166), drew a sharp distinction in the following terms:

> Public ritual behavior asserts something about the *social* status of the actor; private ritual behavior asserts something about the *psychological state* of the actor.

Much of the contemporary cultural critique of 'psychological' therapy seems to accept this distinction and, like Leach and many of his contemporaries, seeks to shift the focus of attention from the latter to the former. But it is worth pointing out that there have always been voices within anthropology that have sounded cautionary notes when it comes to accepting the common sense obviousness of such distinctions. In response to Leach, the Sri Lankan anthropologist Gananath Obeysekere (2014[1981]:14) pointed out the problem that

> for Leach all public symbolic communication is devoid of emotional meaning or psychological content. This position introduces a radical hiatus between public and private symbols, as it does between culture and emotion.

This radical hiatus or split between the public and the private or the cultural and the individually emotional may be useful from certain analytic perspectives, but a moment's reflection will tell us that it is not always a ready-made distinction to be clearly found in our lives or the lives or our informants, clients or patients. It is perhaps no coincidence that Obeysekere was more attentive to the potential pitfalls of simply accepting this distinction as an empirical reality than many of his contemporaries in anthropology, on the one hand, and that he is still best known as an anthropological theorist of psychoanalysis, on the other. His caution that such distinctions are themselves matters of perspective remains valuable at a time when the potential danger is that psychotherapy might correct a one-sided emphasis on a bounded interior with a shift to an equally bounded exterior, leaving aside the vital question of how and why that boundary comes into being from different perspectives (see also Seeley in this volume).

Dependence and interdependence

It may be argued that ultimately even the most 'relational' forms of psychotherapy, such as British Object Relations, ultimately focus on the construction of a kind of bounded individualism as the outcome of successful emotional development or psychotherapy. Hence, even for Fairbairn (2001[1941]:42),

> mature dependence involves a relationship between two independent individuals, who are completely differentiated from one another as mutual objects . . . the more mature a relationship is, the less it is characterized by primary identification; for what such identification essentially represents is failure to differentiate the object. It is when identification persists at the expense of differentiation that a markedly compulsive element enters into the individual's attitude towards his objects. . . . The abandonment of infantile dependence involves an abandonment of relationships based upon primary identification in favour of relationships with differentiated objects.

Emotional maturity would then seem to involve a paradoxical form of 'dependence . . . between two independent individuals'. It is a situation to be distinguished from immature dependence on the basis that it has failed to move beyond the stage of 'primary identification', in which the person has yet to 'differentiate' her own self from the objects to which she is attached. Hence, to an extent one can agree with McLeod, that in this conception healthy functioning does appear to rely upon the maintenance of a boundary between inside and outside and a focus on the internal relations, which are to be distinguished from those that are best experienced as external, even for as relational a figure as Fairbairn. But the construction of that boundary is itself an achievement that grows out of interpersonal relations, between infant and caregivers or client and therapist, to provide just two obvious examples. And this is the case for even the most 'intrapsychic' therapeutic figures such as Freud, for whom the resolution of relational traumas (such as the Oedipus Complex) was the basis upon which persons were ideally formed, and for whom the self was inherently made up of aspects of other persons (such as the super-ego as the manifestation of parental attitudes within the pre-differentiated core of the developing infant's person). Even the Freudian self, allegedly the outcome of purely internally contained drives and essences, only develops in a healthy or pathological direction by virtue of the particular relations that it takes into and expels from itself in the course of its development. Psychotherapy did not simply adopt a bounded individualism but was also characterised by a (sometimes semi-aware) recognition of the relational dependencies upon which that individualism relied (whether it welcomed that individuality or viewed it with some suspicion). This is a tendency that has been made explicit at a number of occasions in psychotherapy's history. The so-called Cultural School in New York in the mid-twentieth century, whose members included Horney, Fromm and Sullivan, provides perhaps the most striking example of the long history of engagement with these issues and concepts within the discipline. Erikson famously had a lifelong engagement with these themes, working alongside anthropologists and directly observing the patterns of childhood interaction in Native American communities in order to build up models that stressed the role of culturally variable relational entanglements in personal development. To this list, dozens more names could easily be added, such as

Laing's controversial analysis of schizophrenia as a response to social relational problems. The key concept in this analysis was the 'double-bind', itself taken originally from research conducted by the anthropologist Gregory Bateson on the *Naven* ritual of New Guinea (see also Krause this volume).

Indeed, what is perhaps most striking about psychotherapy as an example of twentieth century Western thought is the extent to which it strove towards a recognition of the ways in which a full understanding of human being necessitated a constant shifting between perspectives. It focused on the otherwise inaccessible and hidden corners of the psyche, while simultaneously drawing attention to the immense amount of relational work that had to go into differentiating the inside from the outside of the person. Hence the seemingly paradoxical nature of the formulations of some of those who struggled with this dynamic most deeply. The ostensible contradiction of 'dependence' between 'independent individuals' was well apparent to Fairbairn (ibid.), who also spoke of the manner in which in 'infantile dependence',

> the object with which the individual is identified[,] becomes equivalent to an incorporated object, or, to put the matter in a more arresting fashion, the object in which the individual is incorporated is incorporated in the individual.

The work of distinguishing inside from outside is never complete, and Fairbairn seems to suggest that dreams often express not so much repressed sexual urges, but a part of the person that still desires to dissolve that boundary and return to an undifferentiated primary identification. Whether this position is best characterised simply as an expression of a 'bounded individualism' that continues a tendency in Western thought characterised by writers such as Hobbes or Descartes is itself ultimately a matter of perspective. As Scharff and Birtles (2001:xi) note, Fairbairn at points consciously differentiated his approach from the Platonic mind/body dualism that he saw as being too influential in Freud's writings, drawing instead on his studies of other figures within Western thought, such as Hegel and Lotze, who challenge that starting point. Indeed, the ways in which thinkers such as Fairbairn approached these issues suggests that they were in many ways approaching a position that stressed the construction of persons out of relational entanglements; this was in many ways far more nuanced than many of their contemporaries in anthropology, who were largely working within a tradition that stressed the opposition of 'individuals' to 'society', as if the existence and emergence of individuals could be simply assumed.

Of course, it is still possible to critique psychotherapy in general for drawing its boundaries too tightly around what it considers to be important in the relational world. Hence, even with its focus on immediate family relations, Object Relations and other relational approaches in psychotherapy could still be critiqued for ignoring 'wider' social problems leading to mental distress. Again, however, it is worth noting that this is not an entirely new critique. Many figures in the history of psychotherapy, such as Fromm, made precisely this point many decades ago. And even if more explicitly relational forms of psychotherapy can still be subjected to varieties of this criticism, they still show that the root cause of this problem is not as simple as psychotherapy's unconscious attachment to a particular form of bounded individualism associated with a caricature of the orthodox Freudian analysis. Rather, it illustrates the ongoing nature of problematic process by which we draw the boundaries of the unit of analysis, and limiting the chain of relational entanglements from which that unit is formed, whether it be the individual person, the nuclear family, the extended family or 'wider' society or culture as a whole. These objects of analysis are formed in the interactions (such as that between parents and children or therapists and clients), as all objects might be said to be formed as objects of perception through the very process of differentiating them out of the flux of experience from which they emerge.

The rise of culture

Recent years have seen an upsurge of interest not only in 'cultural' therapy but also 'relational' forms of psychotherapy and psychoanalysis more generally. Here psychotherapy mirrors a turn in anthropology and social sciences more generally, in which a long-standing interest in the nature of social relations has been foregrounded and intensified in recent years. In both disciplines, a central focus on social relations as the fundamental building block of persons is a distinguishing feature of many, or perhaps most, leading practitioners.

Historically, British and American anthropology were divided by the former's concentration on 'society' and the latter's focus on 'culture' as their abstractions of choice. Today, both of these models are often critiqued for constructing an image of culture or society as an abstraction that stands separate from the individual and in some way moulds or socialises her. It is this conception that often appears to underpin the 'cultural' models that have been increasingly imported into fields such as provision of public services, public policy, management consultancy and psychotherapy in recent decades. The irony is that within the social sciences, critiques of this framing have become increasingly influential at precisely the same time as they have been taken up outside the academic disciplines that gave birth to them. Authors such as the sociologist Bruno Latour and the anthropologist Marilyn Strathern have been at the forefront of calling into question the assumption of such a thing as 'society', for example. Similarly, a variety of authors in anthropology, most notably those associated with the volume *Writing Culture* published in 1986 (including a contributor to this volume, Vincent Crapanzano), led the charge against the idea of 'culture' as something existing objectively outside of the anthropologist's construction of it in text as an explanatory device. These critiques have a number of different emphases, but they share a common concern, that many earlier models of 'culture' or 'society' were built with the purpose of simplifying and translating messy and ambiguous or contested perspectives on relations and ideology into fixed, stable patterns or structures. This process of cultural simplification was carried out predominantly for Western audiences, first of academics and then of administrators or consultants who needed such a conception of 'society' or 'culture' as a relatively fixed stable entity, shared among its members in order to use it for purposes of public and private management.

In the following discussion of critical engagements with this history, I focus on the work of Marilyn Strathern as an example of an influential anthropological thinker from recent years. Although Strathern has written about the dangers of treating 'culture' as a reified abstraction (see Krause this volume), her focus has been more on the problems inherent in assuming a 'Western' conception of 'society' as the universal shared basis of all human existence. Her critique is among those that most explicitly addresses the issue of relational entanglements as being at the heart of being human, in a manner that presents a useful point of comparison with the history of dealing with similar issues in psychotherapy.

Strathern's critique of the idea of 'society', which had been prevalent in twentieth-century British social anthropology and sociology, is most developed in her most famous book, *The Gender of the Gift*. In this book, she argues that the idea of society as an external force, standing outside of and above individuals and shaping them in particular ways, is itself a peculiarly Western way of thinking about the importance of social relations in people's lives. One can easily find examples of work from previous generations of social scientists that seem to illustrate the kind of perspective that she is holding up for critical interrogation. To provide one example from many that I could present, we can take influential British social anthropologist Victor Turner's description of Ndembu initiation and healing rituals in Africa. Turner (1985[1964]:41) describes them as being processes in which the power of society 'is felt to change, the inmost nature of the neophyte, impressing him, as a seal impresses wax.'

With this conception of an inner core moulded by a socio-cultural power that appears as an external force, it is no wonder that Turner also provides at times an example of the long-standing anthropological tradition of drawing a sharp distinction between 'social'/'cultural' and 'psychological' explanations, to the detriment of the latter, as noted by Davies (this volume). 'Here again a cultural explanation seems preferable to a psychological one', he observes at another point of the discussion (Turner op cit:50). No wonder also, then, that Turner's depiction of Ndembu healing rituals is one of the anthropological texts cited in most detail by McLeod, who also promulgates such distinctions between cultural and psychological explanations, similarly to the detriment of the latter. McLeod (2006:51) describes Turner's depiction of Ndembu ritual in glowing terms as a therapeutic process that is 'highly collectivist' and involves 'all members of the village community'. He compares this favourably with individualised Western therapy where the patient would in all likelihood meet individually with a psychotherapist, and might use his leisure time to consume music and visit the outdoors'.

It is worth noting that this romanticisation of such collective activities might be shared by many members of 'the' community but may well not be so enthusiastically experienced by others who are expected or forced to participate. Indeed, the idea that there is such a thing as 'the' community is one that contemporary anthropological accounts tend to call into question, preferring to ask how it is that membership of a community is ascribed and contested rather than taking it as a given. And the starkness of the contrast between Western individualist culture (bad) and Ndembu collectivist culture (good) would certainly not be shared by many contemporary anthropologists, who would be concerned at how such blunt contrasts might cover up diverse positions and interests within these 'cultures' – normally to the detriment of those with the least power – to assert their vision of desirable cultural values and practices.

Such approaches, based upon the way that 'society' as an external force shapes 'individuals', can also be critiqued for reinscribing the very assumption of 'individualism' that they set out to decentre. For although they place a great deal of determining power on the nature of different socio-cultural structures in human life, they can often assume that society or culture or civilisation emerge to deal with the problems inherently contained within each individual (Freud's monsters from the Id arguably being a fine example). In so doing, they seem to assume that there is a fundamental separation between the innate individually contained core substance of the person and a set of social relations that in some way stands separate from and even opposed to her.

Strathern's project is to a very large extent one of creating a new vocabulary that might enable Western social scientists to move beyond assumptions that she sees as fundamental to concepts such as 'culture' – in particular the conceptual opposition between 'individual and society'. The most important terms in Strathern's lexicon are probably 'relational', 'sociality', 'dividual' and 'partible'. All of these terms push anthropological analyses towards less bounded conceptions of the person in a manner that might bear comparison with the way in which psychotherapy's subject matter has often pushed practitioners in the same direction. The most fundamental conception of 'relational' personhood simply means that relations are the primary defining feature of human being; that persons are constructed out of relations; and that this should be our starting point rather than the conception common in 'Western' thought (as both Strathern and McLeod might characterise it) that individuals and their innate internal drives, desires or capacities are the fundamental starting point. 'Sociality' for Strathern refers to the importance and existence of social entanglements in all aspects of human life, internal and external; it is contrasted to the idea of a 'society', standing separate and outside of the individual person in a necessary but sometimes antagonistic relation to her, that she argues is common in Western political thought.

Strathern's work is particularly closely associated with the concept of the 'dividual' person. She contrasts this with the model of the 'individual' common in Western political thought, which she describes in the following terms:

> Persons receive the imprint of society or, in turn, may be regarded as changing and altering the character of those connections and relations. But

> as individuals, they are imagined as conceptually distinct from the relations that bring them together.
>
> *(Strathern 1988:12–13)*

The tradition that Strathern ('the imprint of society') is referring back to includes such figures as Turner ('impressing him, as a seal impresses wax') and earlier figures in anthropology such as Radcliffe-Brown and his great sociological influence, Durkheim. By contrast, Strathern (op cit:13) argues that the Melanesian people who are the focus of *The Gender of the Gift*

> are as dividually as they are individually conceived. They contain a generalized sociality within. Indeed, persons are frequently constructed as the plural and composite site of the relationships that produced them.

Far from lying outside of them as an external object that they both possess and are shaped by, in the form of society or culture, sociality *is* the 'within' as well as the 'outside' in this dividual conception of the person.

The phrase 'dividual', although today largely associated with Strathern, first appeared in the work of the anthropologist McKim Marriot in his 1976 paper, 'Hindu Transactions: Diversity without Dualism'. In this paper, a similar description of the dividual as a different conception of the person who transcends common oppositions between the internal individual and the external social aspects of life is clearly laid out:

> actors are not thought in South Asia to be 'individual', that is, indivisible, bounded units, as they are in much of Western social and psychological theory as well as in common sense. Instead, it appears that persons are generally thought by South Asians to be 'dividual' or divisible. To exist, dividual persons absorb heterogeneous material influences. They must also give out from themselves particles of their own coded substances, essences, residues, or other active influences that may then reproduce in others something of the nature of the persons in whom they have originated.
>
> *(Marriot 1976:111)*

This in many respects fits the classic cultural relativist template imported into psychotherapy – that a particular kind of non-Western set of people (in this case South Asians, in Strathern's case Melanesians) have a mode of personhood that does not stress individualism, as it might commonly be conceived of. But far from describing these entanglements in terms that imply they take the form of an external 'culture' that stands outside of 'individuals' and then shapes them, here the relations pass in and out of persons in the very process that makes them in the first place. The key task that the concept of 'dividual' then achieves is precisely to dissolve an assumed foundational separation between the pre-social inside and social outside of persons. Instead, all internal aspects of persons are ultimately particular configurations of relations between persons, as Marriot summarises with the claim that, for these dividuals,

> what goes on between actors are the same connected processes of mixing and separation that go on within actors.
>
> *(Marriot 1976:109)*

While the concept of the 'dividual' has gone on to become influential in anthropology via the work of Strathern, it has also been taken up by influential figures in psychoanalysis and psychotherapy, not least the Indian psychoanalyst Sudhir Kakar; Kakar has drawn upon the concept to make sense of the different experience of conducting therapy with Indian clients, who he argues are more likely to see their own person in these dividual terms, while also being keen to stress that, as a cultural dichotomy, its importance and absolute status should not be 'overstated' (Kakar 1982:275).

The final idiom of 'partibility' of persons is obviously a close cognate of those already mentioned. It is fundamentally the idea that aspects of persons (who themselves have been formed out of relations) can be separated out from those persons in order to help form other persons. Strathern quotes Fred Damon's (1980) ethnography of the *kula* gift exchange ceremonial cycle in Papua New Guinea to make the point that 'a person throws away part of himself, his "hand", and this self is only reconstituted as it is used to make other selves' (1980:280). This is part of a wider network of reciprocal relations that Strathern, following Damon, describes as a process for 'the creation of persons' (Strathern 1988:193).

For Strathern, the social problem faced by Melanesians is the creation of persons by differentiating persons from the social relations out of which they emerge, rather than the 'Western' problem of bringing inherently atomised individuals together into a unified entity called 'society'. One can see how this 'Melanesian' conception of how the person is formed bears some comparison with ideas of how a separate sense of self emerges in many psychotherapeutic conceptions. The infant has no sense of self at first and experiences an undifferentiated unity with her environment, most significantly her primary caregivers. Through a long process of introjecting her relationship with those caregivers, she is able to finally construct them, and therefore herself, as a separate person. There are clear differences between these two processes, of course. The former is a very public process in which whole groupings come together to perform this construction of persons through the process of acknowledging their origin, in relations from which they are then differentiated. The latter is often a more private process that the person may remain largely unaware of unless they consciously reflect upon it in a process such as therapy. Therapy can be seen as analogous to ceremonial ritual, then, not in the sense that it imposes the power of 'society' upon 'individuals' (though many people have indeed characterised both processes in this manner), but instead because they could both be viewed as ways in which the processes by which persons are formed out of relations are reflected upon, consciously acknowledged and potentially rearranged.

It is worth reiterating that, once the unfamiliar contexts and terminology are put aside, there should not be too much in this to unduly surprise or unsettle many psychoanalysts and therapists. The idea that parts of persons, or relations with them, become introjected into other persons as the core of the very process by which persons are formed is fundamental in particular to Object Relations but can be seen in most other modalities of therapy as well. Likewise, the idea that a sense of self foundational to the creation of persons is not inherent but has to be built in and out of these relations is not core to Object Relations alone. It is this conception that leads many Gestalt practitioners to view Gestalt as a fundamentally 'relational' theory, for example, despite its common characterisation as the most highly 'individualistic' school of therapy. Generations of anthropologists have denigrated psychoanalysis and psychotherapy for a singular focus on the 'interior' of bounded individuals, and today influential figures within the discipline itself have adopted this critique. But perhaps psychotherapy's legacy might be better characterised as one that has always problematised the distinction between the inside and outside of the self by showing how the same relations make up both, and it is only through a careful process of sorting and differentiation that particular boundaries between the inside and the outside of the self emerge. While anthropology has since the 1980s begun to increasingly adopt versions of this kind of perspective, psychotherapists – beginning with the likes of Rank and Klein – have been moving in this direction under the pressure of their material since the 1920s. Perhaps psychotherapy was always well ahead of anthropology in this regard; if anthropologists (and increasingly contemporary theorists with psychotherapy) were to lose their reliance on 'psychologising' as a quick term of abuse, they might be more open to the possibility that some of the innovations in post-structural and relational anthropology from the 1980s onwards had been prefigured in psychotherapy for decades.

To say that the individual is not a bounded individual entity foundationally separate from and prior to the relations into which it enters is not necessarily to say that there is no self that experiences a difference between its inner essence and an outside environment at all. It might instead mean that we had to begin by looking at how that self was constructed from a process of differentiating between different kinds of social relations and entanglements.

A starting point for analysis might properly be the processes by which such distinctions are drawn, and in particular those processes that seek to make that process an object of conscious reflection (such as ceremonial exchange rituals or psychotherapy) in order to shape its course and the boundaries of the self that is formed from it. Such a perspective would then focus on the way that the self is a shifting, ongoing process of becoming made in relation with others, rather than assuming it is a fixed entity to be worshipped or destroyed. It would suggest a focus on what has always been at the basis of psychotherapy as theory and practice: namely, that the self is painstakingly constructed out of the environment of which it is a part and that the outcome of that process is never be entirely taken for granted as a stable achievement but rather as an ongoing work in progress.

On becoming a person

The process of becoming a person can then be seen to be one of the internalisation and externalisation of relations or relationally acquired capacities and objects. Although rarely explicitly theorised in exactly these terms, the centrality of this process can be seen in both ethnographic and psychotherapeutic accounts. *The Gender of the Gift*, for example, is full of references to such processes. We find at first many references to the already established thesis that, for Melanesians, there is ultimately no distinction between inner and outer essence. But the creation and display of the moving back and forth between inner and outer states still at times remains an important part of how human essence moves between and constitutes persons.

> These Melanesian cases delineate *the impact which interaction has on the inner person*. . . . Consequently, *what is drawn out of the person are the social relationships of which it is composed*: it is a microcosm of relations. . . . Awareness of them implies that they must be attended to. These *internal relations must either be further built upon or must be taken apart and fresh relationships instigated.* The kinds of initiation ritual to which I have been referring stage just the awareness or acknowledgment of the necessity of so taking further action, and of the possibility of doing so.
>
> *(Strathern 1988:131; emphasis added)*

In this description, Melanesian conceptions of the person draw out the realisation that every aspect of the person is composed of social relationships, right down to what Westerners might conceive of as the most irreducibly natural and individually bounded element of the individual person: the human body itself. The construction of this person from relations is never a completed process but instead has to be constantly maintained, with relations that are now 'internal' having to be built upon or dismantled. The purpose of ritual is to bring this process to 'awareness' and to acknowledge the necessity of continuing to attend to it if it is to proceed in a good manner.

Strathern suggests on occasion that an interest in 'boundaries' and their maintenance is an expression of a particular Western conception of a unitary bounded self. Yet although everything is relational and the inside and the outside of the self cannot be distinguished on the basis that one is the location of relations and the other is the location of pre-relational essence, drawing a distinction between inside and outside is on occasion unavoidable. Strathern's own discussion of the impact of interaction on 'the inner person' is just one example. Indeed, what is clear implicitly from Strathern's depiction is the way in which relations and relational objects pass in and out of the person as part of its ongoing constitution.

The 'impact of interaction on the inner person' is balanced by the way that 'the social relationships of which it is composed' are 'drawn out' of it. Or as Fairbairn (op cit:43) might have it,

> the task of differentiating the object [and hence differentiating the self from the object] tends to resolve itself into a problem of expelling an incorporated object, i.e. to become a problem of expelling contents.

Even if Strathern at times appears to be sceptical of boundaries in general, much as McLeod is sceptical at times of 'selves' in general, the very distinction between inner and outer and the depiction of relations and relational objects moving between them suggests that some aspects of the person are impossible to conceive of without some kind of idea of a boundary, both for Strathern and for the Melanesian persons whose experience she is trying to capture. What both the public rituals that Strathern describes and the private ritual of relational psychotherapy mark is an attempt to bring to consciousness and shape that process by which relations are introjected and extrojected from persons who(se boundaries) *are formed by that very process.*

Despite Strathern's suspicion of the idea of a boundary, the movement across an implicit boundary between inside and outside is clearly a central component of Melanesian idioms of personhood as she understands them, as is also illustrated in the following passage, in which she claims that Melanesians

> *locate the sources of their internal efficacy beyond themselves.* The sources do not constitute some other realm or domain but another type of person. . . . These sources are not to be controlled or overcome but sustained in order to give perpetual evidence of this very efficacy. . . . They are perpetually preserved since *they are required* to elicit, in Wagner's phrase, the body's capacities, *to externalize* and make known *its internal composition.* ***But the difference between internal (intrasomatic) and external (extrasomatic) relations has itself to be made known***, and this is done through the imagery of replication, through the collective character of the events by which what is made known about one body is repeated for many.
>
> *(Strathern ibid.)*

Here there is an inner self, but the origin of its capacities is to be found outside of itself. This does not imply that a distinction between inner and outer is unreal or unimportant. On the contrary, the distinction is important, but it is not given or fixed; instead, it constantly has to be 'made known'. Or, as Winnicot (2005[1951]:3) might have it, 'the perpetual human task of keeping inner and outer reality separate yet interrelated'.

Hence, Strathern's descriptions of the ways in which relational essence can be taken inside and moved outside suggests some kind of conception of a boundary, albeit one that is more fluid and constantly made and re-made in practice than a 'Western' one that is either given at birth or ideally fixed at a certain developmental stage (as with classical Freudian psychoanalysis, for example). If the relations that make a person 'are not in a state of stasis' and 'awareness of them implies that they must be attended to' (Strathern op cit:131) constantly, then it would make sense that the same would apply to the boundaries across which relations flow inside and out. Indeed, to attend to the one is inherently to attend to the other. The self that the Melanesian gift exchange ritual seeks to create is not fixed at birth or fixed at a particular early stage of relational constitution, as in Freud's ideal schema. It may achieve momentary unitary status through the incorporation of different relational elements in an ideal balance rather than through their exclusion or repression. Hence Strathern's critique of earlier theorists like Herdt, who, inspired by Freud, saw Melanesian male initiation rituals as the attempt to create unitary males through the expulsion of inherited feminine aspects in order to create totally unitary masculine adults. For Strathern, Melanesian masculinity and femininity are based on the correct balancing of male and female relational elements inside the person, rather than a Freudian scheme that begins from innate bisexuality and progressively represses and then expels the aspects that threaten a unitary adult gender identity. Again, it is worth noting in this regard that in her move away from idioms such as repression and expulsion towards concepts such as balance, praised by the anthropological community as profoundly revolutionary, she is following a path trodden by many post-Freudians within psychoanalysis and psychotherapy, from Rank onwards.

The contents of the book

In many of its psychodynamic and humanist forms, psychotherapy can be seen as a practice designed to improve this process of making persons out of relations by bringing it to awareness and consciously reflecting upon it. To the extent that psychotherapy can be considered an 'individualistic' practice, this is the kind of individualism that it has often promoted. Although aspects of Freud's work do suggest a conception of 'society' as a repressive force that emerges in response to the innately destructive urges contained in all of us, other therapeutic perspectives have long stressed a more relational individualism that is forged out of an awareness of the relations that constitute it, rather than one that constructs those relations as external pressures that appear in the shape of a 'culture' or a 'society'.

The different chapters of this book explore these themes raised by the relationship of anthropology and psychotherapy from different angles. Many chapters explore the meaning of the incorporation of 'culture' into psychotherapy and ask in particular how this incorporation can be understood in terms of a wider context of changes occurring inside the discipline. Davies, Krause and Martin, for example, all discuss the adoption of particular models of 'culture' in the context of changes designed to bring psychotherapy training and practice under increasingly formalised structures of professional oversight. All three authors have a concern with the 'performative' power of language: that is, the power of language not merely to describe a situation but also to shape it or bring it into being. Sociolinguistic discussions of the 'performative' power of language most often use public moments when a change of status is conferred by a particular use of language as examples. 'I now pronounce you husband and wife', 'I arrest you in the name of the law' and so on. But any therapist will be familiar with the process in which 'naming' an emotion does not merely describe it but brings aspects of it to awareness, and in that very process changes the experience of the emotion that it purports to describe. Psychotherapy as a 'talking cure' is an emblematic example of the way in which these performative aspects of language can reshape the nature of the phenomena being described by the speaker, including the subjectivity and selfhood of the speaker herself. This performative aspect of language, which has increasingly come under the spotlight of anthropological investigation in recent years, has been central to psychotherapeutic practice from its inception. It is also a part of the more public process by which particular therapeutic sensibilities and orientations are developed and inculcated in training. A more experienced colleague in the Manchester therapeutic community who trained in a rather orthodox 'Person Centred' establishment in the early 1990s described to me once the ferocity of resistance from trainers if any of the trainees dared to use the term 'counter-transference' to describe aspects of an interaction with a client, even if it seemed to capture important aspects of the relationship. Rogers had clearly stated that the term to use was 'congruence', and the insistence on this term rather than its Freudian alternative was clearly felt to be important to the moulding of a particular 'Person Centred' therapeutic subjectivity (as was the shift from 'patient' to 'client' as well). Today the introduction of 'culture' marks a similarly important shift, and Krause, Davies and Martin use different material to discuss the ways in which 'culture' is used in a performative manner in contemporary therapy practice, training and governance. It is clear that there are a thousand potential different meanings to the term 'culture': its relation to particular ethnicised groups, its relation to individual persons, the extent to which it is seen as being located within or outside of them and so on. How it is used in any particular moment therefore suggests a conscious or unconscious deliberate decision to use the term to create a particular object of intervention in that context. We may be able to find all kinds of justification for doing so, but it is important to remember that these are lines that we choose to draw to justify certain courses of action as much as they are neutral descriptions of distinctions that objectively exist outside of their deployment.

A perspective that focuses on the situated use of the concept of 'culture', most importantly what it does for the person using it in that particular moment, is most associated in anthropology with the theoretical revolution launched by the edited collection *Writing Culture*, published in 1986. One of the key contributors to that collection was Vincent Crapanzano, and in his chapter in this collection, he is also concerned with the performative or pragmatic power of language. Crapanzano's paper is focused predominantly upon the re-exploration of a famous case of analysis: Vincent Binswanger's analysis of Ellen West in Switzerland in early 1921. Crapanzano's focus is on the previously mentioned concept of 'transference'. What work is done by characterising particular relationships and emotions that they evoke as 'transference'? How far can the concept usefully be expanded outside of analytic contexts without losing any explanatory power? The issue of 'culture' raises its head here as well, and Crapanzano joins other authors in expressing concern about 'the dangers in stressing cultural difference in psychotherapy', or at least one might add, the dangers of stressing particular models of cultural difference that imply that they are the shared properties of unified separate groups (see also Martin this volume). It is perhaps hardly surprising that Crapanzano should be so acutely aware of the dangers of this model, as someone who was at the forefront of growing trends to subject this conception of 'culture' to critical interrogation in the 1970s and 1980s and to replace it with a more 'reflexive' understanding of how the concept of 'culture' itself shaped the persons who used it as a device to make sense of their relation to others. This has occurred at precisely the point that the older model it supplanted seems to have been taken up outside the discipline in a variety of fields, including psychotherapy. There is little doubt that Crapanzano's long interest and engagement with psychoanalysis was a key component in his developing interest in the self-reflexive aspects of ethnographic research, forcing the ethnographer to explore her own subject position in her construction of a particular conception of culture rather than presuming that the 'culture' was an object out there to be scientifically described. Given the importance of Crapanzano's work to the development of this perspective, this can be seen as an example of how anthropology has developed by virtue of an often-hidden relationship with psychoanalysis and psychotherapy. The irony is that the hidden nature of this psychoanalytic influence on anthropology means that the critique of the earlier models of culture that it partially inspired is also largely hidden from a trend in contemporary psychotherapy that wishes to simply introject those earlier models wholesale.

Other chapters also tackle the issue of 'culture' head on in a different manner. Seeley's chapter, for example, looks at the role that cultural perspectives might have in helping to understand different generations of traumatised refugees arriving in the US. Like Siddique, her approach is at times more sympathetic to the potential positives of adding 'culture' to therapists' understandings than some of the previously mentioned texts, pointing out the lacunae in understanding that can occur when wider aspects of life-worlds outside of therapeutic explorations of childhood trauma are ignored. Possibly this different evaluation comes in part from working in the USA, as opposed to the UK, where the three therapeutic practitioners previously mentioned (Martin, Davies and Krause) operate and where the compulsory introduction of 'cultural' competencies can be seen as part of a general trend of top-down managerial audit that all three view with some suspicion. It can also perhaps in part be put down to her greater engagement with orthodox Freudian analytic trends that have traditionally had the strongest aversion to discussion of psychic distress in terms other than the repetition of infant traumas within individual adults.

Kitanaka and Siddique's chapters also raise issues of 'cultural' difference. Like McLeod, Siddique draws upon the anthropological work of Victor Turner, raising the possibility that the therapy room might be, to use Turner's term, a 'liminal space'. But although, like McLeod, she is also keen to stress the importance of 'cultural' factors that have at times been discounted in the therapeutic encounter, her framing seems more optimistic about the possibilities for that 'third space' to transcend fixed distinctions between inner and outer worlds or between subjects and their cultures. Similarly, like McLeod, Kitanaka discusses a 'distrust of the psychological' and the desire to rummage in the interior of the person, positing this in the material she discusses as possibly being to an extent a reflection of particular tendencies in wider Japanese society. She cites authors who also critique the idea of the Freudian self as being uniquely Western and bounded from a Japanese perspective. But as an anthropologist, rather than wishing to take that critique simply at face-value, she seeks to explore the interests behind its promotion and the inevitable downsides of such depictions of 'cultural selves' with regard to their potential erasure of differences to do with class and gender *within* particular 'cultures'. One of her concerns is that caricatured romanticisations of the Japanese communal self are simply constructed in opposition to an equally one-sided caricature of the Western. In this regard, she shares the concern of many anthropologists with models that continue to promote this kind of generic cross-cultural comparison. Kitanaka's chapter illustrates the ways in which different conceptions of the self to be explored in therapy emerge not as the expression of a shared essential cultural code but through historical processes involving factors as complex as changing patterns of healthcare funding and responses to natural disasters.

What the chapters in this collection all show is that the current adoption by psychotherapy of a model based on 'cultural competence' is only one way in which the idea of bounded individual selves in therapy might be deconstructed. Indeed, a more sympathetic reading of the history of psychotherapy might suggest to us that psychotherapy itself has consistently pulled at the threads of bounded individualism in manners that might be in some regards more enlightening than the particular model of culture that some in psychotherapy seek to import from previous generations of anthropological research. They certainly demonstrate that the potential for the two disciplines to learn from each other has many more potential avenues to explore than this one and that the development of a continuing dialogue between them should not be limited to the promotion or rejection of the current 'cultural' agenda.

References

Damon, F. (1980) The Kula and Generalised Exchange: Considering Some Unconsidered Aspects of the Elementary Structures of Kinship. *Man*. n.s. 15:267–292.

Fairbairn, R. (1941[2001]) A Revised Psychopathology of the Psychoses and Psychoneuroses. In R. Fairbairn (ed.) *Psychoanalytic Studies of the Personality*. New York: Taylor and Francis.

Kakar, S. (1982) *Shamans, Mystics and Doctors: A Psychological Inquiry into India and Its Healing Traditions*. New York: Knopf.
Leach, E. (1958) Magical Hair. *The Journal of the Royal Anthropological Institute of Great Britain and Ireland*. 88(2):147–164.
Macpherson, C. (1962) *The Political Theory of Possessive Individualism: Hobbes to Locke*. Oxford: Oxford University Press.
Marriot, M. (1976) Hindu Transactions: Diversity without Dualism. In B. Kapferer (ed.) *Transaction and Meaning*. Philadelphia: ISHI Publications (ASA Essays in Anthropology 1).
McLeod, J. (2002) Lists, Stories and Dreams: Strategic Invitation to Relationship in Psychotherapy Narrative. In W. Patterson (ed.) *Strategic Narrative: New Perspectives on the Power of Personal and Cultural Stories*. Lanham, MA: Lexington Books.
McLeod, J. (2006) Counselling and Psychotherapy as Cultural Work. In L. Hoshmand (ed.) *Culture, Psychotherapy and Counseling: Critical and Integrative Perspectives*. Thousand Oaks: Sage Publications.
Obeysekere, G. (2014[1981]) *Medusa's Hair: An Essay on Personal Symbols and Religious Experience*. Chicago: University of Chicago Press.
Scharff, D. and Birtles, E. (2001) Introduction. In R. Fairbairn (ed.) *Psychoanalytic Studies of the Personality*. New York: Taylor and Francis.
Strathern, M. (1988) *The Gender of the Gift: Problems with Women and Problems with Society in Melanesia*. Berkeley: University of California Press.
Turner, V. (1985[1962]) Betwixt and Between: The Liminal Period in Rites of Passage. In A. Lehmann and J. Myers (eds.) *Magic, Witchcraft, and Religion: An Anthropological Study of the Supernatural*. Palo Alto: Mayfield Publishing Company.
Winnicott, D. (2005[1951]) Transitional Objects and Transitional Phenomena. In D. Winnicott. *Playing and Reality*. Abingdon: Routledge.

1

LESSONS FROM THE ANTHROPOLOGICAL FIELD

Reflecting on where culture and psychotherapy meet

James Davies

An auto-ethnographic introduction

Like an ethnographer perpetually shifting between two cultures, for the last twenty years I have spent my professional life moving in and out, through and between the distinct life-worlds of social anthropology and psychotherapy. By the time I first became interested in anthropology in my early twenties, I had already spent two years undergoing psychotherapy myself as well as some years reading psychotherapy literature in an attempt to further understand myself, others and the psychotherapeutic process I was passing through. In particular, I read representative works in therapeutic traditions such as the analytic/relational (S. Freud; D. W. Winnicott; H. Kohut); the cultural (K. Horney; E. Fromm; H. S. Sullivan); the humanistic (C. Rogers; F. Pearls; A. Maslow); and the analytical psychological (J. Hillman, S. Jeffers; C. G. Jung). In fact, it was the more anthropologically informed writings of the latter school, and in particular the deep cultural preoccupations of Carl G. Jung, which helped me gravitate to social anthropology when choosing my undergraduate degree.

Enrolling at the School of Oriental and African Studies in the late 1990s, I embarked on what turned out to be an intensely post-structuralist education, replete with French relativistic and American post-modernist thought. What arose as a consequence was entirely unexpected: a thorough recalibration of the broadly individualistic and internalising psychotherapeutic *weltanschauung* I had previously adopted. Those formal studies unexpectedly changed my relationship to therapeutic ideas. I no longer regarded them as more or less scrupulous depictions of reality but as cultural artefacts, ideological supports, or social responses, liberating or enslaving, depending on whom and by whom they were used – as bearing, in short, a social life of their own. Ideas, for me, now fell from their glittering sphere of objective revelation to join that earthily panoply of cultural phenomena ripe for anthropological analysis. My intellectually naivety had passed, and much psychotherapeutic lore, including my attachment to it, was demystified as a result.

While many psychotherapeutic ideas had for me lost much of their potency (at least as totalising explanatory tools), the notion that psychotherapy could be a useful social practice remained robust – something evidenced by my decision, after graduating in anthropology, to begin formally training as an adult psychotherapist. Once I had put this decision into effect, however, new and unanticipated problems soon arose. The highly critical and expository culture that I had become familiar with as an undergraduate was now supplanted by what felt like an asinine vocational training that taught us, in almost seminarian fashion, what to believe and what to do, without requisitioning any inquiry into the social construction of belief and action. I soon learned that the critical atmosphere of my anthropological training was less welcome in the therapeutic academy. And internal tensions ensued as a result.

As such tensions would soon only escalate, I decided to place my psychotherapeutic training on hold to pursue graduate studies in social and medical anthropology, which, after encountering for the first time many fascinating works in psychological and psychiatric anthropology, culminated in my writing a dissertation on the nature of psychotherapeutic belief: what enabled psychotherapists, in the post-metanarrative era, to make an almost modernist commitment to operate within a set mode or schema of thought – to defer and maintain faith in a mode or practice that was, after all, under increasing sceptical onslaught? In particular, I became interested in what role professional socialisation played in deflecting powerful post-modern headwinds: in preserving an enclave of decided belief and practice where the newly initiated, upon accreditation, could find a secure professional, moral and ideological home.

Such questions underpinned my decision to pursue my anthropology doctorate on essentially the socialisation of psychotherapeutic professionals, largely focusing on persons and institutions within the psychodynamic/psychoanalytic tradition. With my supervisor's support, I therefore took up my psychotherapeutic training again, but this time as both trainee and ethnographer – becoming a psychotherapist while at the same time studying this process of becoming anthropologically. My therapeutic training became part of my field site – my peers, patients, therapist and trainers, my informants. My oscillations between the two traditions, previously swaying languidly between distant points, now pitched and veered ever closer – almost to vibration.

My qualifying as a psychotherapist in the very same month I submitted my anthropology PhD on psychotherapeutic socialisation symbolically signalled the comingled world I would come to inhabit: a coterminous life that still lives on. Within three months of qualifying, I had begun my first university lectureship – this time largely teaching, it transpired, anthropological insights to psychotherapeutic trainees. Within twelve months my anthropology doctorate had been published by a psychotherapy publisher (Davies 2009) and was therefore being mostly read by psychotherapists. Within three more years I was now also lecturing in anthropology. Two years later I had taken up a full-time anthropology readership. For the past seven years I have continued teaching, practicing, supervising, researching and writing within both disciplines, in what at times feels like either a protracted season of fieldwork or a prolonged therapeutic relationship with anthropology on the couch.

The upshot of this alloyed position has been my distanced-affinity for both traditions. Like a child pulled by parents at cross-purposes, I inhabit a compromise somewhere in-between. Perhaps a similar sense of liminality is what Vincent Crapanzano recently referred to when saying he has 'always felt tangential to the [anthropological] field . . . always tangential to everything' (Crapanzano 2015). Most anthropologists will understand this sentiment, whatever the admixture of variables from which their marginality is hewn – professional, ethnic, religious, political. But perhaps fewer will share this feeling with respect to the homeliness of their own discipline, feeling sometimes comfortable, sometimes not.

The above is more than mere biographical indulgence. It provides the context out of which my absorption in the relationship and interplay between anthropology and psychotherapy has dominated my professional life: one I have expressed through exploring how anthropology and psychotherapy, broadly defined, are and can be creatively and mutually informing. Whether using psychotherapeutic ideas to inform anthropological practice (e.g. in the domain of fieldwork; Davies and Spencer 2010), using anthropological theory to understand facets of psychoanalytic culture (e.g. the transmission of psychoanalytic knowledge; Davies 2009) or integrating both perspectives in the study of any social or human phenomenon (e.g. emotional suffering; Davies 2011), I have perpetually struggled to work at the interface, attempting to chisel spoils from that space in-between.

The argument

In what follows, I shall continue in that effort, this time by bringing anthropological insights to bear on a central theme of this current volume – how the concept of 'culture' as it is currently used guides or misguides contemporary therapeutic theory, training and practice. My aim in this chapter is to scrutinise anthropologically a growing trend within contemporary therapeutic provision, especially with respect to how culture should be understood, managed and responded to in the therapeutic setting. My aim is to articulate a series of propositions, informed by anthropological theory but broadly inconsistent with today's increasingly manualised psychotherapeutic trainings, whether such trainings operate in universities or through NHS/IAPT initiatives or private training institutes. My argument is that, apart from in some specialist anthropologically informed corners, such as the Nafsiyat Intercultural Therapy Centre, manualised psychotherapeutic training, which aims to attain consistency in results and conations across practitioners, has in this pursuit become increasingly culture-blind. Not through failing to articulate a concern for culture, or as is usually put, cultural difference, but through having become wedded to a concept of culture as something *possessed* – as something one *has*, rather than as something one *does*.

When consulting the relevant literature on culture and psychotherapy, in recent years there has been a shift toward foregrounding the development of 'cultural competency' as an essential matter in training – whether that training occurs in standard counselling work (Ahmed et al. 2010); IAPT-based CBT (Bassey and Melluish 2012; Department of Health 2011; NICE 2011); or long-term therapeutic work (Stanley et al. 2009; Tummala-Narra 2016). This narrative largely frames cultural competency as the capacity to negotiate skilfully the cultural differences existing between members of the therapeutic encounter – i.e. developing cultural 'sensitivity' to dissimilarities of 'language', 'concept', 'behaviour', 'perception' etc., in view of facilitating practitioner understanding and a deeper therapeutic alliance (Collins and Arthur 2010). The dominant assumption of the cultural-competency narrative, in other words, is that culture resides *in* practitioners/client/patients – in persons who *have* culturally rooted responses and reactions, which interact, intermix, clash or cohere with those of others. What matters in any consideration of culture, therefore, is developing competency in negotiating these interactions, differences and embroilments in service of understanding, through the deployment of a cultural skill-set absorbed through one's specialist training.

While the competency narrative may, in important ways, both highlight and help people better navigate difficulties encountered in the process of negotiating difference, I argue that the institutional move towards a focus on developing 'cultural competency' has a flipside by concealing a powerful ideological shift away from considering *therapy itself* as a work of culture, as an embedded culture practice on its own terms (Furedi 2004; Seeley 1999; Klienman 1988; Littlewood and Kareem 1992; Smail 2001; Luhrmann 2001). Rather, culture, from the cultural-competency standpoint, is increasingly configured as a thing *possessed* by clients and therapists, as something with which and on which therapy works. This subtle splicing of culture from practice to persons, from something one *does and enacts* as an outcome of therapeutic acculturation, to something one *has* in the most colloquial sense, wrongly elevates therapy above that with which it works, and in consequence denies persons-in-practice certain vital ways of thinking about the work they do.

What I shall therefore argue is that the vision of culture assumed by the competency narrative is at variance with an almost axiomatic principle in social anthropology: *that practice is culture*, and that by extension therapy is profoundly context making and thus constitutes, when exercised on trainees and clients/patients, a highly specific form of acculturation. My aim here is to offer a series of propositions through which to explore the notion that therapeutic practice is culture enacted: propositions to be illustrated by way of previously unpublished ethnographic material gathered from fieldwork largely undertaken in 2007.

The materials pertinent to this current chapter derive from six months' participation in clinical group supervision as a participating psychotherapeutic practitioner. These weekly sessions comprised three trainee psychoanalytic psychotherapists, one consultant psychiatrist and one psychoanalytic group facilitator, all of whom worked within a context where cultural competency was expected from practitioners. These sessions thus provide a useful context in which to analyse cultural-competency strategies at work. With respect to other observations made in this chapter about the state of training today, these are derived from my role in the community as practitioner and therapeutic educator; from anthropological fieldwork carried out in the psychotherapeutic community between 2003 and 2005; and through many subsequent ethnographic 'fieldwork expeditions', to use Emily Martin's (2009) phrase, that my professional role in the therapeutic community habitually affords.

Proposition one

Therapeutic nomenclatures (theoretical, diagnostic) are just as much proscriptive (i.e. context creating) as they are explanatory and descriptive (i.e. context referring) – culturally scripting how suffering is understood, managed and thus experienced.

I wish to illustrate the above proposition by way of some general reflections on the diagnosis of mental health problems. I choose not to use the term 'psychiatric diagnosis' because over the last thirty years, mental health diagnosis has ceased to be only used by psychiatrists and is increasingly used by a wide array of psychotherapeutic, counselling and mental health professionals. In the NHS today, people cannot access mental health/psychological services without first undergoing a diagnostic test (Johnstone and Watson 2017), obliging diverse mental health professionals to work and think within a common medicalised diagnostic framework. The proliferation of diagnostic thinking across mental health provision is now reflected in the number of psychotherapeutic trainings, of differing modalities, teaching the rudiments of diagnostic thinking and practice or else legitimising the diagnostic act (Johnston 2014). While these trainings may differ in the extent to which they acknowledge the culturally constituted nature of diagnostic categories (these categories, after all, are not rooted in any known biomedical markers), and while also they differ in the extent to which they acknowledge certain adverse effects of diagnosis (i.e. social and self-stigma it can generate), there are still certain effects of diagnosis passed over in most clinical and training contexts today. To aid facing these squarely, let us consider the following ethnographic vignette. Here, I present to my peer-supervisory team a case study concerning my therapeutic work with a 30-year-old man:

> During group supervision I report to the team that Patient X, who had a diagnosis of bi-polar disorder, suggested to me in our previous therapeutic session that other patients in the psychiatric day centre, sharing the same bi-polar diagnosis as him, were often playacting. They would receive the diagnosis, and then begin to exaggerate the relevant symptoms

> and behaviours deemed characteristic of the condition. He surmised that this probably occurred because they would read up on their condition after being diagnosed and then adapt to what they read. Other patients, he noticed again and again, were becoming *more* bi-polar after being so labelled. He was adamant this kind of subterfuge was going on widely in the NHS, and was baffled why doctors seemed largely oblivious to it.

When discussing this matter with the supervisory team, the professional response was to doubt Patient X's perceptions. Even if some instances of subterfuge did occur, this behaviour was surely not as widespread as Patient X alleged. Was Patient X becoming paranoid? Was he somehow envious of other sufferers? Was he trying to impress himself as the only authentic patient? What, in essence, were the psychodynamics of his assertion? While such lines of enquiry may be expected in a supervisory context, it was never considered that Patient X could in some sense be correct: that the people he observed were indeed becoming *more* bipolar after their diagnoses were issued, a phenomenon that has been noted elsewhere in the ethnographic record (Martin 2009). When we inquire as to why this possibility was not considered, we espy the work of certain assumptions about diagnosis at play: in particular, the idea that diagnostic categories essentially *describe* emotional and behavioural states. While this view is pivotal in diagnostic manuals such as ICD and DSM, as well as permeating various diagnostic tools widely used in training and practice (e.g. PHQ9 and GAD7), it of course obscures a central component of diagnostic labels: that they are highly *proscriptive* cultural symbols, helping shape and direct the forms of suffering they purport to disinterestedly describe.

To verify the proscriptive effects of diagnostic labels, ample ethnographic and epidemiological data have revealed how such categories pattern and shape suffering in both its collective and individual forms. With respect to collective suffering, for example, we know that when new descriptive categories take hold of a group, they can direct how it experiences and expresses its suffering. This fact has been richly illustrated by work analysing the stigmatising effects of diagnostic labels (appellations which, by medicalising suffering, radically influence how it is socially perceived, managed and experienced [Pirutinsky et al. 2010; Corrigan and Watson 2002; Johnston 2014; Goffman 1963]) but also by work revealing how new disorder categories, having become accepted and reified in that group's imagination, alter the course emotional distress can take (Shroter 2013; Hacking 2002; Harrington 2012; Lakoff 2004; Skultans 2003; Watters 2011).

To illustrate this latter dynamic, consider for a moment the issue of 'mental disorder' epidemics and the interesting fact that when a new disorder is introduced to manuals, such as DSM, incidence rates of that disorder regularly escalate. For example, after Attention Deficit Hyperactivity Disorder (ADHD) entered DSM-IV in 1994 (replacing the previous ADD), rates tripled by 2004 (Frances 2013); after Dissociative Personality Disorder entered the DSM in 1980, related cases rose from 200 to 40,000 over twenty years (Maldonado and Spiegel

2008); after Bipolar II was added in 2000, the ratio of bipolar versus unipolar depression doubled by 2010 (Frances 2013); and after self-harm entered the DSM in 1994 (as a symptom of 'Borderline Personality Disorder'), instances of self-harm doubled in ten years (Whitlock et al. 2009; Davies 2013).

Within the mental health community, the most common explanation for the above escalations is that once a disorder is recognised by the DSM, doctors are more likely to look for it in their patients, patients are more likely to look for it in themselves and pharmaceutical companies are more likely to market the condition and the relevant medications. While of course such factors may help account for these escalations in part, they can by no means be considered exhaustive. As the work of Hacking (2002) and Shroter (2013) has shown, once a new disorder becomes accepted by a given cultural group, it often begins to act as a novel expressive possibility, providing a new cultural script in terms of which persons may now recite their distress.

An apposite anthropological term for this scripting of suffering would be 'mimesis' – the process by which people unwittingly absorb and perform shared cultural scripts about how to act in order to achieve certain desired ends. It is well documented in the anthropological literature that mimesis regularly occurs in the performance of distress, enabling the communication of suffering through ways-of-being that are socially recognisable (Romberg 2009; Harrington 2012; Skultans 2003; Taussig 1993). In short, human beings seem to be invested with a developed capacity to mould their bodily and mental experiences to the norms of their cultures, or, as Anne Harrington has put it, 'to learn the scripts about what kinds of things should be happening to them as they fall ill . . . and then they literally embody them' (Harrington 2012). After all, it is crucial we express our distress in ways that make sense to the people around us; otherwise, we will end up not just ill but ostracised (ibid.). Thus understood, the notion of mimesis is heuristically useful in explaining why the ratification of new disorder categories can increase incidences of the very phenomena they purport to depict.

To illustrate how the above idea can also fruitfully elucidate certain day-to-day particulars of the clinical setting, I would now like to return to our opening ethnographic vignette and, chiefly, to the accusation Patient X levelled at certain other patients diagnosed with bipolar – namely, that they were often playacting. One important question arising here could be whether Patient X was correct to level this accusation, or whether the team was correct to regard his accusation as a symptom of his 'illness'? However, in light of our above discussion of mimesis, this either/or question now seems to miss the point, as it entirely overlooks that diagnosis can be *proscriptive*. In other words, when we allow for the proscriptive nature of diagnosis, a third interpretative possibility arises: that the bipolar patients accused of subterfuge were simply enacting mimesis unawares – unwittingly reciting the bipolar script to which their diagnosis had newly introduced them.

As soon as we entertain this new perspective (i.e. that conscious subterfuge and unconscious mimesis can look remarkably alike), the entire supervisory event assumes a different meaning: Patient X now appears correct to accuse others of imitation (but mistaken in believing it was calculated), while the supervisory team appears correct to question Patient X's perception (but mistaken in pathologising it). These mistakes occurred because neither party fully appreciated the extent to which diagnostic labels proscribe experience. Instead, their interpretations stem from the traditional assumption of descriptiveness: an assumption bleaching cultural agency from the diagnostic system itself. As a result, culture is seen as rooted in those who either issue or receive a diagnosis, rather than in a system whose facility to shape experience (i.e. transform it through description) is clear to all those analytically disposed to see.

What is illustrative about the above case study is that while no obvious cultural-competency work was practiced by the team (the issue of 'cultural differences' never arose), cultural work certainty transpired in this setting; culture, after all, was given a specific location – in persons and not (diagnostic) systems. This kept all participants walking the well-travelled paths of perception that guide practice down familiar routes.

Proposition two

Psychotherapeutic systems bring to the facts the philosophies they claim to derive from them, contrary to what it taught.

Psychotherapists are often taught, although not always explicitly, to operate as though the therapeutic thought-styles into which they are initiated can, at their very best, generate accurate insights into the 'clinical' phenomena encountered (Davies 2009; Luhrmann 2001; Loewenthal 2011). Such conviction in the power of therapeutic systems to capture the true mechanics of psychological experience is no doubt bolstered by a growing disinclination in many trainings to teach and learn psychotherapeutic systems as situated works of culture that lose efficacy to the extent they lose cultural legitimacy (more so, in fact, than the other way round). The following clinical vignette will help us tease out some clinical correlates of this proposition:

> In clinical supervision a colleague reports on his work with Patient A, a 45-year-old, female, first-generation Greek immigrant, who identifies as Greek orthodox. He reports how his therapeutic relationship with Patient A is in tatters. We are told that despite his numerous attempts to help her confront how her early trauma was relevant to her current troubles (her father died when she was eight), she rejected this line of inquiry as irrelevant to her current depression and her struggles with her teenage son. The therapist claimed that the ensuing impasse with Patient A explained the patient's loss of faith in therapy, her increasing insistence that therapy wasn't helping, and her growing desire to terminate their work.

The response of the supervisory team was to suggest the therapist slow down. Perhaps he had forced the interpretation too early; perhaps Patient A was resistant 'for understandable cultural reasons' to the idea early trauma could do lasting harm; maybe the therapist could try to explore the breakdown in therapy so as to repair it – exploring culturally rooted beliefs around the notion of trauma, loss and death. It was agreed that the therapist could have handled this better, being more mindful of the cultural mechanics behind Patient A's response to the early loss of her father. The consensus arose that Patient A's relationship to trauma, as well the therapist's inclination to force the interpretation, should be examined more deeply.

Structurally speaking, the above supervisory move is fairly typical. The team locates the cause of breakdown between therapist and Patient A within both parties: in the therapist's poor interpretive timing and/or in Patient A's resistance. Here, the team uses the very psychological system of meanings rejected by Patient A to explain her and her therapist's behaviour. This move has implications for both parties insofar as it effectively de-legitimises Patient A's protest by suggesting her dissent is for reasons other than she states (not because, as she thinks, the therapist is wrong, but because, as they think, she is afraid or resistant); while at the same time it affirms the therapist's narrative, which, by pathologising Patient A's doubt in therapy, deflects doubt from the system itself.

Any anthropologist familiar with the literature on the management of therapeutic failure or rupture will recognise the structural underpinnings of the above interpretative move. Long before Karl Popper advanced his ideas on falsifiability, as early as 1937 Evans Pritchard coined the term 'secondary elaboration' to describe how the Azande doctor he observed protected the oracle's power by blaming instances of failure on anything other than the oracle itself (Evans-Pritchard 1977:124) – a move also noted by Tanya Luhrmann in her analysis of therapeutic mishaps among witchcraft rituals in North London (Luhrmann 1989:253), and by Elisabeth Hsu in her reflections on failure within Chinese traditional medicine (Hsu 1999:52). All such systems betray a common (i.e. structural) response to therapeutic failure, insofar as all regard systems failed by way of selves, either through being resisted (by recipients) or misapplied (by practitioners) – moves which, by rooting all failure in persons, effectively render the system unfalsifiable (Davies 2009).

Some years ago, I informally surveyed how far psychotherapeutic trainees had embodied such structural responses by asking ten at random how they accounted for failure in their therapeutic work. Of those questioned, only one admitted to sometimes doubting the applicability of a certain idea to a given case, while the remaining nine made comments such as: 'I would look to the relationship and ask what had occurred between us to sabotage our work'; 'you can never entirely blame the patient, there is always something you could have done differently'; 'some patients might not be ready for depth analysis, this should always be considered'; and 'a therapist must always be ready to question what they have missed' (Davies 2009). While psychoanalytic practitioners made the above statements,

I more recently repeated the same exercise with those training in the tradition of CBT. I was interested to find the same kind of secondary elaboration at play: the cause of failure being rooting within either the therapist or patient and thus deflected from the system itself.

Returning now to our above vignette, what such management of perceived failure may teach us is that the insights psychotherapeutic systems generate are less exact apprehensions of reality than logical consequents of viewing the world through a particular therapeutic lens. What this means, in clinical terms, is that these systems often bring to the clinical facts (including the facts of failure) of the philosophies they claim to derive from them. While this may sound fairly obvious to the relativist (i.e. that theorising itself is a more or less useful form of cultural practice), to ignore it means a host of alternative interpretative moves are logically silenced as viable possibilities – those that would allow for, in this instance, an entirely different response to the case of Patient A.

To contextualise the above in the light of earlier reflections on cultural competency, the performance of 'competency' by the above supervisory team could be read euphemistically as an act of 'secondary elaboration'. What 'cultural competency' amounts to in this case is locating failure within the culture of persons and not the system enacted. And so here we witness secondary elaboration being performed in the name of cultural competency, insofar as such competency is exercised to preserve and defend a fairly predictable style-of-thought with its accompanying tranche of interpretative strategies. To the supervisory team, alternative strategies simply do not arise as possibilities for consideration, owing to the absence of any working framework through which they can be entertained and explored. The irony here is that in the absence of such a framework, many relevant social dynamics remain unavailable or 'unconscious' to the team; or, in other words, that 'unconsciousness' does not stem from avoiding the embrace and application of therapeutic knowledge but *only* from embracing and applying therapeutic knowledge.

Proposition three

Therapeutic change is due to non-technical factors (i.e. symbolic/ structural/ common), rather than to technical factors (i.e. processual/specific).

Let us explore this proposition by returning to the previous vignette, re-joining the team's deliberations about Patient A three months after we left the above scenario. By now, the previous breakdown in the relationship has been repaired. The team believes this was triggered, in part, by the therapist recommending a book to Patient A on the effects of trauma and loss (an unorthodox move, perhaps, but one endorsed by the team). Following this, Patient A failed to attend the next two sessions, only to return a week later with a new conviction that her father's death was indeed relevant to her current suffering. Over the next two months her commitment to therapy increased, something also expressed by her joining an online loss/trauma discussion group. Furthermore, her mood also improved. We pick up group supervision at this more sanguine phase in therapy:

> The therapist reports that, despite these changes, Patient A's husband had become suspicious of her new reading material. Last week the husband had found a therapy book and hidden it, and also declared, during an argument, that she was being 'brainwashed'. The therapist reflected that the husband's hostility seemed to be growing proportionately to Patient A's deepening commitment to therapy and, more meaningfully, to the easing of her depression.

The supervisory team is careful not to accept Patient A's depiction of events uncritically (was she displacing her own lingering resistance to therapy onto her husband, using him as a proxy for her criticisms?). They also reflect that the husband's response, if taken at face value, could potentially subvert the therapeutic work. Considering his charge of brainwashing, the team sympathises that the husband feels threatened by the evident changes in his wife. They also reflect on his 'traditional Greek Orthodox view' of the role of a wife and mother. They suggest the husband/wife relationship be further explored in therapy, paying careful attention to these cultural dynamics and also noting that Patient A's previous hostility to her therapist may have been transferential. Finally, the supervisory team interprets the improved therapeutic alliance as vindicating their earlier interpretation of why therapy broke down (due to Patient A's 'resistance' and/or the therapist's lax therapeutic technique). It is agreed that the maintenance of a strong therapeutic relationship will be essential in protecting Patient A from any further challenge her husband may advance.

From the supervisory team's perspective, what they see as therapeutic progress is also believed to have stemmed from the fruitful deployment of a suite of interventions and meanings – resistance, interpretation, transference, trauma, rupture – that repaired the therapeutic alliance. In essence, we observe the team, to use Arthur Klienman's (1988) terms, identifying factors *specific* to the psychotherapeutic process as responsible for therapeutic change, rather than factors broadly *common* to diverse healing systems. As the distinction between the *specific* and *common* factors is useful in unpicking key dynamics in the case of Patient A (and as it is rarely discussed or even recognised in the psychotherapeutic settings I have observed), I believe a brief description is necessary before our analysis can proceed.

From the 1960s onwards, research into what has been called 'equivalence' had a seminal effect on the psychotherapeutic profession. This research showed that when different psychological therapies are compared, they all broadly perform equally well or 'equivalently', assuming the same amount of contact time between patient and therapist (Luborsky and Luborsky 1975). What appeared to shape outcomes was less the mode of therapy deployed than the quality of the relationship developed between therapist and client:

a theory that has been broadly asserted ever since (Roth and Fonagy 2006; Flückiger et al. 2012).

*

From the 1980s, many anthropologists came to agree that the quality of the therapeutic relationship was integral to success. Additionally, they used the findings of 'equivalence' as a spring board to identifying other common drivers of efficacy that operated in a whole array of therapeutic systems cross-culturally, psychotherapeutic or otherwise (Dow 1986; Kleinman 1988; Calestro 1972; Prince 1980). This work broadly asserted that efficacy was unrelated to the very specific technical transactions and rationalisations that individual therapies deploy. Rather, efficacy emerged from the evocation of powerful cultural symbols, which appeared to influence persons through their 'meaning effects' (Moerman and Jonas 2002). For example, while 'therapeutic allegiance' (i.e. a shared belief in and enthusiasm for therapy) and 'patient expectation' (i.e. shared expectation recovery will happen) are both noted to be key drivers of efficacy (Blease and Kirsch 2016), for allegiance and expectation to occur at all presupposes the existence of a therapeutic explanatory system (a system of symbols and meanings) in which both parties can place their faith. For such systems to be worthy of faith, however, anthropologists like Kleinman argued that they must provide a convincing 'symbolic bridge' between personal experience and the wider socio-cultural world (1988). When an explanatory system aligns with a wider field of credible cultural symbols (e.g. medical or political symbols), this bridge siphons credibility into the system itself, boosting the 'allegiance' and 'expectation' of its adherents (and thus therapeutic outcomes), while at the same time enabling the patient to integrate into that wider social field of symbolisation (i.e. as the symbolic bridge gives private experience public orientation, the straying individual is reconciled with the social whole).

Interestingly, much of this anthropological work referred to such explanatory systems as 'mythic' systems (Dow 1986), because it was not essential whether such systems were objectively true (i.e. whether they revealed psychological 'reality' so to speak), rather whether they held experiential truth for their users. It was from the act of believing in their potency to heal that most of their efficacy was gained (Davies 2009). In short, long before more recent studies revealing the powerful placebo effects of psychotherapy (Blease and Kirsch 2016), anthropologists have been documenting how such common symbolic factors allow healing expectations and allegiances to crystallise (Moerman and Jonas 2002); a perspective helping us to account for why diverse systems can be equivalent in outcome when they profess such different myths, meanings and protocols.

*

The purpose of discussing the above is to shed light on the aforementioned case study, as it offers us a different theoretical prism through which to read the events. For example, we recall that a key concern of the supervisory team was the husband's accusation that Patient A was being brainwashed by therapy. While the team interpreted this as the husband feeling threatened by the change his wife was undergoing, it never considered whether the husband has a legitimate cause for concern, which is theoretically possible from the standpoint of the symbolic perspective discussed above. For instance, as Patient A gradually acclimatised to a new set of meanings regarding the most intimate features of her subjective life (new meanings to which she was becoming emotionally attached), the husband interpreted this as a process of conversion: his wife adjusting to an explanatory system unfamiliar to his own, an adaptation generating not just subjective effects for her but also social effects for her immediate group.

So, what were those social effects? The clue is found in noting that at this point in therapy, Patient A had yet to experience the social dislocation that seeing the world differently to her husband and family subsequently introduced: an effect of therapy that is well documented in the anthropological literature, and one which soon impacted Patient A after the said events. As soon as we allow for this effect, the husband now seemed to be responding to a dimly sensed nascence of this dislocation. His protest, in other words, was less a spasm of cultural chauvinism than of anxiety at how his wife's conversion would alter perennial family relations and structures. What the team perceived as a movement towards health, he perceived as a threat to familial integrity. What the team read as remedy, he alternatively read as the onset of new malady (social dislocation).

The reason why malady was interpreted as remedy becomes clear when we assume the symbolic perspective: as the supervisory team witnessed the patient's improvement, they put this down to the specific healing powers of therapy rather than to more common symbolic factors (e.g. as therapist and patient became evermore woven into a shared web of symbols and meanings, this mutuality boosted the expectation of recovery, and thus the outcome). The ascription of healing to the *specific* healing factors of therapy, then, not only betrays a certain self-interested interpretative bias but also poses a potential hazard: if we ignore that healing often occurs for reasons other than our therapies profess, our relationship to those therapies becomes distorted – deferential, over-reliant and uncritical: all things wielding palpable clinical effects.

When we relate these points to our earlier reflections on 'cultural competency', this phrase, once again, seems to almost act ideologically. Insofar as the team acted with 'cultural competence' in this case, the phrase merely characterises a form of sensitivity to the cultures of those involved *in* the therapeutic encounter, while circumventing the culturally situated system of meanings *framing* the encounter. Where we actually locate culture through our conceptualisations, in other words, is essential to what we regard as culture, and thus to what is perceived as the proper material for so-called cultural-competency work.

Discussion – intentionality

What my involvement in these and many other therapeutic sites has taught me is that socio/cultural interpretations of clinical material are rarer than often supposed in the therapeutic community. In one respect this is understandable – psychotherapists are not explicitly trained to think socio/culturally, just as surgeons are not taught to administer the anaesthetic. But we must be careful not to reduce the matter of bounded thinking to a simple deficit in anthropological education. There are stronger forces of motivation and intention at play, ones difficult to dislodge via mere changes to curricula. In short, what I am alluding to is an almost structurally fortified resistance to the performance of certain forms of socio-cultural thought in therapeutic contexts – a resistance built into the habitus of the system itself, and one reinforced by professional socialisation. I am of course not the only commentator to have made this observation – the critical psychotherapy literature is replete with similar claims (Loewenthal 2011; Smail 2001; Gellner 1985; Furedi 2004). And the arrow does not point in only one direction – the term 'psychologism', after all, is still used pejoratively by some British social anthropologists to designate anyone who would presume to use psychological ideas in service of socio/cultural analysis.

Given the various tensions existing between the anthropological and psychotherapeutic traditions, I would like to spend the final part of this chapter briefly inspecting the differences out of which theses tensions may arise. I shall do this by going beyond the more obvious differences in practice, concept, method etc., to inspect what I would call the *different modes of intention* that underpin the psychotherapeutic and anthropological enterprises, using the word 'intention' to refer to the aims and purposes (both inferred and declared) of those operating within a given domain of social practice. What I am interested in are less the specific intentions of individual actors (which are always confounded by diverse idiosyncratic variables), but in what John Searle has called the 'collective intention' – namely, the commonest set of intentions collectively formed and obtaining within a specific social group.

To try and identify collective intention is a perilous task, liable to interpretive bias, over-generalisation and over-simplification. Nonetheless, if some general closing reflections are to be offered, I would broadly characterise the main features of anthropology's collective intention as follows: challenging ethnocentrism, de-pathologising and democratising difference, upending reductionism, contesting dogmatism (religious, political, economic, biological), fostering tolerance and cultural understanding, dislodging stereotypical thinking and, of course interrogating power differentials, their supporting myths and structures and their attending effects on diverse and often disempowered groups. These ethical and intellectual intentions are, of course, also political, directly or by implication – ethnographic immersion, after all, transforms the ethnographer's perceptions, beliefs and understandings not only during the process of learning culture but also through the knowledge attained via such transformations, the social spaces to which this knowledge is disseminated. To put it in Malinowski's words, anthropologists intend to liberalise minds, both their own and those of the communities to whom they distribute their knowledge. While the extent to which they achieve this is mutable, and while the involvement of other variables cannot be predicted in advance, these intentions nevertheless broadly obtain as ones at least enjoying collective recognition.

When turning to the collective intentions of psychotherapists, we immediately encounter a very different suite of recognised aims. While anthropological intentions directly or indirectly endeavour to facilitate wider socio-cultural understanding and/or change, psychotherapeutic aims are more particularistic and, I would even say, redemptive in nature. As research indicates, it should not surprise us that the commonest motivation given for training in psychotherapy is the desire to help individuals in distress, and additionally, that most people choosing psychotherapy as a means for helping others do so owing to some kind of previous engagement with therapeutic perspectives as a way of helping themselves (Davies 2009). Like in so many practices with a redemptive programme at their heart, in other words, subjection to the practice can lead to advocacy of the practice – or at least, in those who want to help others, the intention to enact and advocate a practice that has helped oneself.

As my own ethnography of psychotherapeutic training laboured to indicate (Davies 2009), fostering this redemptive tendency as well as spirit of advocacy is central to many modes of psychotherapeutic training. Not only do trainings ensure that those entering the profession are already favourably disposed to the collective intention (e.g. by obliging all trainees to undergo surreptitious vetting in the form of pre-training therapy), but they also ensure its consolidation by way of the pedagogical devices trainings deploy. My research revealed that trainings are places where persons are socialised to uphold and disseminate the values and beliefs of the particular modality into which they are being initiated: places where contesting the modality is often subtly resisted by shrouded institutional devices that mostly work furtively to discourage or penalise dissent. In short, psychotherapeutic training operates in a manner more vocational than critical, in that it generally aims to deepen, rather than undermine, faith and confidence in the modality one is being trained to advocate.

What I am suggesting here is that different collective intentions of anthropology and psychotherapy not only entail significant consequences for how both disciplines engage with the world (as the discussion of the three propositions partly illustrated), but also for how they engage with each other. For example, such differences in intention I believe can assist in explaining the imbalance so often observed in psychotherapeutic and anthropological relations. While anthropologists have a long history, certainly in the United States, of engaging psychotherapeutic ideas in the service of their intentions (either as an object of criticism or as explanatory tool for socio/cultural analysis), psychotherapists have been comparatively resistant in learning and/or applying anthropological ideas. It is almost as if the situating, relativistic and critical occupations of the anthropological enterprise (certainly as it was shaped during the post-structuralist period) are sensed as potentially threatening to the deep cultural and emotional attachments psychotherapists invariably form to their respective modalities (both through their personal experience and professional socialisation): attachments that are not only thought essential to establishing a secure clinical base, but that also serve to advance the interests of the modality itself, largely by emboldening members to engage competing modalities for resources in an increasingly crowded market of 'treatments'. In other words, the psychotherapeutic intention to help others, oneself and to secure or advance one's modality, has not always sat well with anthropology's critical focus on how healing traditions work, gain and secure social ascendency and at what wider social cost. Where these reflections may be deemed important is in helping us explore how this clash of intentions may have mitigated anthropology's impact on psychotherapy, precisely because the insights of socio-cultural enquiry, when applied to the psychotherapeutic enterprise, threaten to weaken attachments to the dominant styles of thought and practice fostered in training and believed essential to the realisation of collectively recognised psychotherapeutic aims.

Where anthropology can be of most service, then, is not only through helping clinicians work better with culture, but by illuminating the ways in which the traditions to which they adhere are themselves cultural forms. Embracing this simple yet often resisted idea can act to liberate styles of psychotherapeutic thought and practice from a certain rigid faithfulness, by inviting scrutiny of the cultural and thus relative nature of these narrative forms. While some may well see this rejection of literalism as a rejection of therapy, we should remember that the value (or otherwise) of any healing discourse has only very rarely had anything to do with whether or not that discourse was objectively true. To see relativism as compatible (even indispensable) with successful clinical work is therefore as old as psychology itself. If the truth of any system, as William James noted, is less rooted in its declarations than in the consequences of belief in those declarations, then we are right to take a pragmatist approach.

References

Ahmed, S., Wilson, K. B., Henriksen, R. C., Jr., & Jones, J. (2010) What does it mean to be a culturally-competent counselor? *Journal for Social Action in Counseling and Psychology*, 3 (1): 15–22.

Bassey, S., & Melluish, S. (2012) Cultural competence in the experiences of IAPT therapists newly trained to deliver cognitive-behavioural therapy: A template analysis focus study. *Counselling Psychology Quarterly*, 25 (3), 1: 223–238.

Blease, C., & Kirsch, I. (2016) The placebo effect and psychotherapy: Implications for theory, research, and practice. *Psychology of Consciousness: Theory, Research, and Research*, 3 (2): 105–107.

Calestro, K. (1972) Psychotherapy, faith healing and suggestion. *International Journal of Psychiatry*, 10: 83–113.

Collins, S., & Arthur, N. (2010) Culture-infused counselling: A fresh look at a classic framework of multicultural counselling competencies. *Counselling Psychology Quarterly*, 23 (2): 203–216.

Corrigan, P. W., & Watson, A. C. (2002) The paradox of self-stigma and mental illness. *Clinical Psychology: Science and Practice*, 9: 35–53.

Crapanzano, V. (2015) Lifetime Achievement Award Lecture. *Society for Psychological Anthropology*. https://vimeo.com/146152809 (accessed 9 December 2017).

Davies, J. (2009) *The Making of Psychotherapists: And Anthropological Analysis*. London: Karnac.

Davies, J. (2011) *The Importance of Suffering: The Value and Meaning of Emotional Discontent*. London: Routledge.

Davies, J. (2013) *Cracked: Why Psychiatry Is Doing More Harm Than Good*. London: Icon Books.

Davies, J., & Spencer, D. (2010) *Emotions in the Field: The Psychology and Anthropology of Fieldwork Experience*. Palo Alto: Stanford University Press.

Department of Health (2011) *Analysis of the Impact on Equality of Talking Therapies: A Four Year Plan of Action*. www.gov.uk/government/uploads/system/uploads/attachment_data/file/213766/dh_123995.pdf (accessed 10 August 2017).

Dow, J. (1986) Universal aspects of symbolic healing: A theoretical synthesis. *American Anthropologist*, 88: 56–69.

Evans-Pritchard, E. P. (1977[1937]) *Witchcraft, Oracles, and Magic among the Azande*. Oxford: Oxford University Press.

Flückiger, C., Del Re, A. C., Wampold, B. E., Symonds, D., & Horvath, A. O. (2012) How central is the alliance in psychotherapy? A multilevel longitudinal meta-analysis. *Journal of Counseling Psychology*, 59: 10–17.

Frances, A. (2013) *Saving Normal: An Insider's Revolt against Out-of-Control Psychiatric Diagnosis, DSM-5, Big Pharma, and the Medicalization of Ordinary Life*. London: HarperCollins.

Furedi, F. (2004) *Therapy Culture: Cultivating Vulnerability in an Uncertain Age*. London: Routledge.

Gellner, E. (1985) *The Psychoanalytic Movement*. London: Blackwell.

Goffman, E. (1963) *Stigma: Notes on the Management of Spoiled Identity*. Englewood Cliffs, NJ: Prentice Hall.

Hacking, I. (2002) *Mad Travellers: Reflections on the Reality of Transient Mental Illnesses*. London: Harvard University Press.

Harrington, A. (2012) *Being Human: Individual + Society & Morals + Culture*. http://fora.tv/2012/03/24/Being_Human_Individual__Society__Morals__Culture (accessed July 2015).

Hsu, E. (1999) *The Transmission of Chinese Medicine*. Cambridge: Cambridge University Press.

Johnstone, L. (2014) *A Straight Talking Introduction to Psychiatric Diagnosis*. London: PCCS Books.

Johnstone, L., & Watson, J. (2017) Just Listen to Their Stories. *Therapy Today*, 28 (3): 30–32.

Klienman, A. (1988) *Rethinking Psychiatry: From Cultural Category to Personal Experience*. New York: Free Press.

Lakoff, A. (2004) The anxieties of globalization: Antidepressant sales and economic crisis in Argentina. *Social Studies of Science*, 34: 247–269.

Littlewood, R., & Kareem, J. (eds.) (1992) *Intercultural Therapy: Themes, Interpretations and Practice*. Oxford: Blackwell Scientific Publications.

Loewenthal, D. (2011) *Post-Existentialism and the Psychological Therapies: Towards a Therapy without Foundations*. London: Karnac.
Luborsky, L. B., & Luborsky, S. (1975) Comparative studies of psychotherapy. *Archives of General Psychiatry*, 32: 995–1008.
Luhrmann, T. (1989) *Persuasions of the Witch's Craft*. London: Blackwell.
Luhrmann, T. (2001) *Of 2 Minds: The Growing Disorder in American Psychiatry*. New York: Borzoi Books.
Maldonado, J. R., & Spiegel, D. (2008) Dissociative disorders. In *The American Psychiatric Publishing Textbook of Psychiatry*, 5th Edn, eds. Hales, R. E., Yudofsky, S. C., & Gabbard, G. O. Arlington, VA: American Psychiatric Publication, 665–710.
Martin, E. (2009) *Bipolar Expeditions: Mania and Depression in American Culture*. Princeton: Princeton University Press.
Moerman, D. E., & Jonas, W. B. (2002) Deconstructing the placebo effect and finding the meaning response. *Annuls of Internal Medicine*, 136 (6): 471–476.
NICE (2011) *Common Mental Health Problems: Identification and Pathways to Care*. www.nice.org.uk/guidance/cg123/chapter/1-guidance (accessed July 2016).
Pirutinsky, S., Rosen, D. D., Shapiro, S. R., & Rosmarin, D. H. (2010) Do medical models of mental illness relate to increased or decreased stigmatization of mental illness among orthodox Jews? *Journal of Nervous Mental Disease*, 198 (7): 508–512.
Prince, R. (1980) Variations in psychotherapeutic procedures. In *Handbook of Cross-Cultural Psychology: Psychopathology*, ed. Draguns, H. C. Boston: Allyn and Bacon.
Romberg, R. (2009) *Healing Dramas: Divination and Magic in Modern Puerto Rico*. Austin: University of Texas Press.
Roth, P., & Fonagy, P. (2006) *What Works for Whom? A Critical Review of Psychotherapy Research*. London: Guildford Press.
Seeley, K. (1999) *Cultural Psychotherapy: working with culture in the clinical encounter*. New York: Jason Aronson.
Shroter, E. (2013) *How Everyone Became Depressed: The Rise and Fall of Nervous Breakdown*. London: Oxford University Press.
Skultans, V. (2003) From damaged nerves to masked depression: Inevitability and hope in Latvian psychiatric narratives. *Social Science and Medicine*, 56 (12): 2421–2431.
Smail, M. (2001) *The Origins of Unhappiness: A New Understanding of Personal Distress*. London: Robinson.
Stanley, S., Zane, N., Hall, G. C. N., & Berger, L. K. (2009) The case for cultural competency in psychotherapeutic interventions. *Annual Review of Psychology*, 60: 525–548.
Taussig, M. (1993) *Mimesis and Alterity: A Particular History of the Senses*. London: Routledge.
Tummala-Narra, P. (2016) *Psychoanalytic Theory and Cultural Competence in Psychotherapy*. New York: American Psychological Association.
Watters, E. (2011) *Crazy Like Us: The Globalization of the Western Mind*. London: Robinson Publishing.
Whitlock, J. L., Purington, A., & Gershkovich, M. (2009) Influence of the media on self-injurious behavior. In *Understanding Non-Suicidal Self-Injury: Current Science and Practice*, ed. Nock, M. Washington: American Psychological Association Press, 139–156.

2

OVERCOMING MISTRUST OF THE PSYCHOLOGICAL

A history of psychotherapy in Japan

Junko Kitanaka

Introduction: Japanese critiques of psychoanalysis

Despite the early introduction of psychoanalysis from the 1900s, psychotherapy in Japan has had a troubling history, characterized by critiques and dismissal from dominant neurobiological psychiatrists, internal battles among psychotherapists, and a prevailing suspicion among the public toward intrusions into the deeply private realm of the individual. As Naoki Fujiyama, the twenty-second president of the Japanese Society of Psychoanalysis, lamented in 2010, psychoanalysis has utterly failed to take root in Japanese society (Fujiyama 2010:175). While psychotherapists have often proven to be popular as writers for general audiences, their actual practice remains meager: though some form of so-called psychotherapy is practiced in hospitals (discussed below) and is covered under national health insurance, psychotherapeutic training is far from systematic and only weakly developed in medical school. Doctors who want to learn psychotherapy often learn on their own or join like-minded others. Although Japanese doctors have engaged with some forms of psychotherapy since the 1900s, and have developed academic associations, even those who show affinity to it have tended to strongly criticize psychoanalysis itself. Their criticisms address heavy reliance on language, rationality, and culturally bound understandings of family and its pathologies (see Doi 1990). What particularly stands out, however, is a persistent caution against inducing psychological insight. For instance, in a 2014 book on basic principles of psychotherapy, Shozo Aoki, a prominent psychiatrist and highly respected psychotherapist, and Kayoko Murase, an influential psychotherapist and the president of the Association of Certified Clinical Psychologists, discuss the importance of not pushing patients to psychological insights through verbalization. They write that therapists have to be wary of the implicit ideal that exposing one's hidden thoughts and desires is a sign of having established a trusting relationship (Murase & Aoki 2014).

Indeed, Japanese psychiatry has been vocal and fertile in construing astute critiques of Western psychoanalysis and proposing indigenous concepts and alternative approaches. Heisaku Kosawa, Japan's first psychoanalyst, questioned the Oedipus complex as a product of the Judo-Christian tradition of a paternalistic family and instead proposed the "Ajase Complex" derived from Indian mythology, where family conflicts center around an all-loving, ever-forgiving, and suffocatingly powerful mother (a theme later elaborated by an influential Jungian Hayao Kawai in his discussion of Great Mother) (Okonogi 1982; Kitanaka 2003; Harding 2014). Masatake Morita, who studied psychoanalysis at Tokyo University because of his own neurosis, came to reject Freud and proposed that the Western obsession with rational self-control is what constitutes neurosis. He created Morita Therapy, the ideal of which lies in "letting go of self-control" and "accepting things as they are," echoing the Zen Buddhist notion of Enlightenment (Morita 1998). The end of World War II and the subsequent American occupation temporarily brought an avalanche of psychoanalytical ideas into Japan, prompting Yushi Uchimura, then professor of psychiatry at Tokyo University, to declare opposition to Freud and what many Japanese psychiatrists critiqued as his "pseudoscience" (Uchimura 1954). While there continued to be a small number of psychiatrists interested in psychoanalysis (usually triggered by their training in German psychopathology), psychoanalysis served more as a tool of cultural critique than a form of clinical practice. Thus, even after it gained some prominence, particularly during the vehement antipsychiatry movement from the 1960s on, psychoanalysts like Takeo Doi, who became professor of psychiatry at Tokyo University in 1971 and helped popularize some of psychotherapeutic ideas in Japan, similarly critiqued the Freudian notion of the self by arguing that interdependency, not individual autonomy, is at the core of what it means to be a person. Doi's insistence on intersubjective, unbounded, and situation-oriented selves now resonates with postmodernist assertions that have since deconstructed the ideal of the Freudian, psychoanalytic self as a rational, logical, and autonomous being (Doi 1973, 1990; also see Mauss 1985; Kirmayer et al. 1998). Yet, such assertions of "cultural selves" have also been critiqued by scholars of Japan as well as cultural psychiatrists as homogenizing and essentializing, erasing differences of gender, class, regionality, etc., and generating what is only a mirror image of an equally false, essentialized notion of the "Western self" (e.g. Mouer & Sugimoto 1986). Some point out how "culture" essentialized in such ways does more harm than good, as it might derail clinicians who are otherwise highly sensitive to complexities and individual differences (Kleinman 1991; Borovoy forthcoming).

As these cultural(ist) ideas seem, by now, dated and faded, and they are necessarily not what Japanese psychiatrists cite when they talk about psychotherapy in their daily practice, what do Japanese doctors actually do in their "psychotherapeutic" practices? What do they mean when a practitioner uses psychotherapeutic methods, and what do they strive towards? These are the questions I had in the 2000s when I conducted fieldwork at a prestigious university hospital that attracted doctors interested in psychopathology, phenomenology, and psychotherapy. This department was headed by a grandson of a pioneering social psychiatrist in Japan, who had a large following for his evocative writings on religion, creativity, and social pathology. A highly respected leader in otherwise biologically oriented Japanese psychiatry, he oversaw the revised translation of Freud's collected works and offered seminars in which psychiatrists and philosophers gathered together to read texts by Kant and Lacan in their original German and French. Creating an intellectually stimulating atmosphere, he led discussions on philosophical and phenomenological meanings of mental illness, providing lecture series with topics that ranged from genetics to Wittgenstein. Psychiatrists offered various therapeutic selections to patients, including individual psychotherapy, group therapy, collage therapy, painting therapy, and music therapy, and discussed both neuroimaging and patients' art works in case conferences. So I was all the more surprised when I heard these doctors mention the interdiction against insight-inducing psychotherapy especially for depression, which was the focus of my study at the time. This interdiction, as I found, certainly had an economic basis, as it was nearly impossible to do proper therapy when doctors regularly see over 40 patients per day and had to sacrifice precious time saved for research to do an hour-long therapy session (which some certainly did). It was also clinical and ethical, however, as they discussed how urging patients to delve into the meaning of their illness would often prolong an ailment and cause other complications (for details, see Kitanaka 2012). In order to explore what psychotherapeutically minded doctors do mean by "psychotherapy," then, I want to examine the trajectory of Japanese psychotherapy, beginning with the influence of two great Japanese thinkers and practitioners, Hisao Nakai and Joji Kandabashi, whose books line the desks of virtually every aspiring psychotherapist in Japan. First, I discuss their ideas and how they reflect what I saw in everyday clinical practice. Second, I point out their strengths and limitations, how even their influence might be waning given new economic pressures on psychiatry, and also how there are alternative psychotherapeutic movements that give new meanings to their legacy. Third, I discuss what I would like to call the "psychiatrization of the lifecycle" and emerging interest in the psychotherapy for old age (with a focus on dementia), which might bring about further innovations in psychotherapy in Japan.

Hisao Nakai

Hisao Nakai is a Renaissance man who is fluent in several European languages and has received numerous awards, including one from the Greek government for his translation of Greek poetry. Along with translating 32 books, including a series of works by Harry Sullivan as well as Henri Ellenberger's *The Discovery of the Unconscious*, Judith Herman's *Trauma and Recovery*, and Allan Young's *Harmony of Illusions*, Nakai himself has written more than 40 books on wide ranging topics, including a definitive book on the history of Western psychotherapy. Originally trained as a scientist in virology, Nakai wrote in 1963 an astute criticism of the Japanese medical system before he switched to psychiatry (Nakai 2010). Bringing his scientific observational skills to his psychiatric clinical practice (or what he calls "participant observation," drawing on Sullivan's work), Nakai carefully investigated the natural history of schizophrenia, with a focus on its onset and recovery process, at a time when people with this illness were socially abandoned in hospitals with little hope for recovery and/or discharge (Nakai 1982a). He established the *Journal of Psychiatric Treatment*, pioneered art therapy by inventing "Landscape Montage Technique" as a diagnostic/therapeutic tool, and later became an ardent promoter of *kokoro no kea* (care of the heart/mind/soul), helping to establish psychological intervention for PTSD on a national basis. Featured in a best-selling nonfiction story titled "Therapist," written by a prominent novelist (Hazuki 2014), Nakai has become synonymous with psychotherapist in Japan, embodying the kind of clinical approach Japanese psychiatrists feel comfortable calling their own – though it might not look much like "psychotherapy" to someone used to insight-inducing practices.

Nakai is an interpreter of maladies par excellence. Perhaps because he himself has had physical illnesses that required hospitalization, and also because he has had many close friends afflicted with mental illness, Nakai maintains that it is mere luck that he has escaped what his patients suffer (Nakai 1983). His ability to "tune in" to patients' experiences stands in sharp contrast to the psychopathological approach popular in Japanese psychiatry in the 1960s–1970s, when doctors often engaged in aggressive verbal interrogation as a scientific means of unveiling the essence of psychoses. Instead of objectifying and verbally dissecting the patient, Nakai, with the sensibility of a poet, translates patients' psychotic experiences in a manner that broadens the scope of clinical empathy. He talks about what it's like to sense the slightest, faintest, and farthest sign with utmost intensity, how exhausting it must be to live with an anticipation that something dreadful would soon happen while having an inexplicable sense of yearning for that something at the same time (Nakai 1979). He observes how patients are constantly pulled and pushed among (counter)forces towards recovery and pathology, between hope and fear, being drained in the process (Nakai 1982a). He would caution doctors against outright denials of delusion as lacking courtesy. Using his training in virology, he has created minutely sketched graphs, documenting all the events, experiences, and feelings that a person with schizophrenia goes through so as to understand both the natural progression of the disease as well as the multiplicity and plasticity of such an experience (Nakai 1982a, 1982b). By capturing the dynamism of psychopathology without freezing patients in Otherness, and prioritizing what he calls "moderate indirectness" as a clinical stance (see Saito 2015a), Nakai has elevated reflexive, empathic listening to a new level of scientific understanding, while painting possible paths towards recovery. Asking what hinders recovery, Nakai has also cautioned himself not to write about particular patients, reflecting on how such an act creates an ambition on the part of the clinician, introducing an element of desire and control that would not be healthy in a doctor–patient relationship (Nakai 1982a:333).

Nakai's psychotherapeutic sensibility largely comes from his ability to historically contextualize patients' illness experiences. In *Schizophrenia and Human Species*, Nakai engages with evolutionary psychiatry to reflect on the significance of schizophrenics, who may have been able to detect the slightest signs of danger and warn others of imminent risk (Nakai 1982b). In "Diligence and Ingenuity as the Ethic of Reconstruction," Nakai traces the origins of depressive personalities in Japan to the rise of a Japanese work ethic during what he calls the "Industr*ious* Revolution" in the seventeenth century (Nakai 1976). In "Theories of Therapeutic Cultures," he examines the sudden flourishing of Japanese religious cults at the turn of the twentieth century, the leaders of which were often desperate women driven to the edge before declaring themselves deities during a psychotic trance and attracting the destitute caught in the social upheaval of modernity (Nakai 1983). He brings a broad perspective to daily practice, showing how to understand the experience of ordinary people driven to mental illness against the forces of history. In paying visits to patients' homes, he attends to geo–historical–political location, building/spatial structure, noise level, interpersonal tensions, and family conflicts that create a specific milieu in which patients have had to cope. From this perspective, he aims to transform not the person him/herself but rather the "milieu that creates an illness by changing various parameters" in such a way as to decrease the patient's burden so that s/he can "float" (see Saito 2015a). Doctors influenced by him talk about how they learned not to focus on "hidden conflicts" and "true desires," but rather on the "situation" in which patients live, so as to lighten the burden, shame, and self-blame that patients often feel about their ailment (Saito 2015a:69). One colleague discusses how he began to pay attention to the rhythm of patients' local lives, and how this led seemingly chronic and apathetic patients to tell him surprisingly rich and vivid stories about their family's fruit farm, brewing of sake, seasonable festivals, and local elections – stories that helped them achieve self-(re)integration (Hirosawa 2015:82–83). Nakai's emphasis on "situation" – and his respect for the ordinary and the mundane – is at the core of what Japanese psychiatrists have come to regard as "psychotherapeutic."

Nakai has also actively combined Western biomedicine with traditional medicine, generating "dialogic psychotherapy through antipsychotic medication" (Kuroki 2015:78). Coming into psychiatry after gaining his doctorate in virology, Nakai writes he was shocked to find what little time psychiatrists spent observing patients when their theories offer so little to go on. While regarding daily clinical practice as a site of examining hypotheses, he has also adopted traditional medical approaches that provide more minute observational skills and therapeutic devices to complement psychiatric consultation. He has learned to take a patient's hand to feel the pulse, check their tongue, facial tone, hair shine, nail color, dampness of palm, and coldness of toes. He asks patients about their feeling when waking to ascertain the rhythm and quality of their sleep (Nakai

1982a). Nakai's therapeutic approaches are also meant to sharpen patients' reflexivity and bodily sensibility as a means of empowerment: he asks patients how medication tastes and feels, drawing on the traditional medical idea that pills that agree with one's constitution taste slightly sweet (a claim criticized by more evidence-based doctors: Saio 2011). Having experimentally taken various kinds of antipsychotic drugs himself (a practice common among psychiatrists of his generation), he warns doctors about how frightened patients often are, worrying that pills might fundamentally alter their being. Thus, it is all the more important that doctors become self-conscious about exactly how, when, and why they should use medication and avoid prescribing it as a means of rendering patients into submission. He compares words to radiation, writing that there seem "to be safety limits for exposure to others' comments and gaze." "Words," he says, "can provide harmful disconnection, repetition, and compulsion, which at times serve to consolidate and degenerate a symptom" (cited in Saito 2015a:70). Thus, it is all the more important that the body should serve as a kind of intermediary for doctor–patient communication, as something interactive and intersubjective, and to be synchronized with (Okubo 2015:73).

Joji Kandabashi

Another psychotherapist who is widely read, along with Nakai, is Joji Kandabashi. Though the two are often in dialogue with and deeply respect each other, their styles are radically different. While Nakai was a professor of psychiatry at Kobe University, Kandabashi left Kyushu University as an associate professor after training young doctors there and started practicing at a hospital in the southern part of Japan, where he now attracts desperate patients from all over the country. Trained by Masahisa Nishizono, the thirteenth president of the Society of Psychoanalysis, and John Hunter Padel at Tavistock Institute in London, Kandabashi is deeply committed to psychoanalysis. He has produced over 32 books, mainly on psychotherapy, many of which have become best sellers, and is constantly invited to give lectures, perform public diagnostic sessions, and provide open supervision at medical schools, hospitals, and clinics all over Japan, where he continues to surprise clinicians with his instantaneous and astute diagnostic skills and therapeutic efficacy (see Fukuoka kodo igaku kenkyujo 1997, 2007). At the same time, he often appears as a trick star, playing with contradictions, evoking paradoxical images, and performing a distinctive mixture of techniques derived from traditional medicine and folk/alternative therapies. Some of his techniques seem "occult" and like throwbacks to the time of Mesmerism, which would either make Freud marvel at Kandabashi's ingenuity or more likely turn over in his grave. Ignored by dogmatic psychoanalysts, Kandabashi's style has caused a heated debate among younger psychiatrists about whether he is a charismatic healer or a mere fraud. In his daily clinical practice I observed, however, he shows little of the flashness that he exhibits in public performances and appears to be a genuinely caring doctor, unlikely to give up on a patient regardless of how difficult a case may be. All of his techniques are attempts to explore ingenious ways to respond to the desperate pleas of those who come to him as the last resort. Indeed, it is this medical commitment that has won the respect of many prominent doctors, including Shigenobu Kanba, the highly esteemed president of the Japanese Society of Psychiatry and Neurology, who praises him for his experimental spirit in formulating hypotheses and discovering novelties in everyday clinical practice (Kanba 2014:106). It is also with his scientific spirit that Kandabashi has confronted psychoanalysis, trying to ascertain exactly where and why it has failed and to explore how to make it more therapeutic.

Kandabashi's rebellion against psychoanalysis was crystalized in a 1974 paper on the danger of excavating secrets (Kandabashi 1988). There was a debate at the time among leading psychotherapists in Japan about the value of "uncovering" and "opening up the heart." In response to a prominent therapist who preached this doctrine, Doi opened fire by critiquing the Western psychoanalytic obsession with revealing pathogenic secrets. He pointed out that there is an implicit expectation that a therapist's job is to excavate and reveal secrets such as unconscious desires, anxieties and conflicts thought to be deeply rooted in childhood experiences. He instead argued for the therapeutic value of kept-secrets by discussing *himitsu* (secret), originally a Buddhist term referring to esoteric knowledge and hidden truth not easily attained (Doi 1972). Doi further cautioned therapists with regard to the fundamentally abstruse nature of self-knowledge and the pervasive sense among lay Japanese that there is something sacred about the inner self that doctors should not carelessly intrude upon. This caution was something that Kandabashi, an ardent practitioner of psychoanalysis at the time, took to heart. Doctors who have long known him tell me of his early days when Kandabashi was surrounded by disciples all dressed in T-shirts and jeans just like him. They were so deeply influenced by him and convinced that he was able to see through them that some of them would get into traffic accidents after just one of his supervisions. His patients often became psychotic after his sessions, prompting him to write, in 1965, his first academic paper on transference psychosis (Kandabashi 1988). Realizing his destructive power, he was searching for ways to "naturalize" psychoanalysis when he responded to Doi's criticism. Kandabashi thus further elaborated on how to advise (particularly psychotic) patients to keep their own secrets to themselves as a way of protecting their self-boundedness, asserting that such social withdrawal would encourage self-growth (Kandabashi 1988 [1974]; cf. Corin & Lauzon 1992). Kandabashi's paper, which defines psychological secrets as an essential element of a healthy sense of self, while largely ignored by psychoanalysts, became an instant sensation in psychiatry more broadly (Araki 1997:3), resonating with rising criticisms about the serious side effects of psychotherapeutic intervention.

In addition, Kandabashi, ever obsessed with words, has called attention to how words create reality (Kandabashi 1984, 1990). Starting his career with people with borderline personality disorder, Kandabashi soon realized how psychoanalytic terminologies – and scholarly Japanese translations for them – evoked an aggressive, confrontational atmosphere. He argued that using words like *resistance* and *defense mechanism* might induce in therapists a desire to break down that imaginary barrier between patient and therapist, when in fact psychotherapy should offer a nurturing space that helps a patient as if s/he were a plant trying hard to bud in an adversarial environment (Kandabashi 2004:142). To cultivate a different set of images, he proposes reframing psychological processes as abilities through such constructions as "ability to shut down emotion," "ability to act out," "ability to rationalize," and "ability to project" (Kandabashi 2004:104). Reminding therapists of patients' struggles, he calls attention to the fact that symptoms are expressions of a patient's power for natural healing – a way of settling with their inhospitable environment – but that their "natural" or first way of being is not necessarily "positive" or the best mode of adaptation. In order to encourage patients to experiment with new modes of being, Kandabashi urges therapists to consciously select three types of words. These are: bodily words (or those that evoke bodily and affective memories), which penetrate deeply into a person's physical being (including the sounds one makes when nodding as well as the sound of silence); abstract words, which have a detaching or calming effect; and parodies, which help destabilize the logical structure that binds the patient (Kandabashi 2004:267–268). In countless open supervisions he has offered, Kandabashi has demonstrated to groups of therapists how he experiments with a gradation of possible expressions, ranging from the dictatorial to the empathic, calling attention to how slightly different wording drastically changes an implicit message and immediately transforms mood and atmosphere. Noting the power of words and images in such ways, he has constantly urged all doctors to choose words that heal, that would aid patients in becoming observers and experimenters of their own mind/body. Kandabashi's attempts also energized the growing psychoanalytic movement from the 1970s to indigenize psychotherapy, as doctors became aware that certain emotion/value-laden words (like *amae*, which often signals pleasurable interdependency; Doi 1973) cannot be easily translated into European languages and that therapists should use vernacular Japanese to achieve genuine understanding.

Kandabashi's emphasis on the body is pushed to the extreme (Kandabashi 1999, 2011). In treating people with severe borderline personality disorder, he recounts how he felt helpless with words, as they seemed to do so little with people who had been hurt at the "preverbal level" (such as those with attachment disorders, who lack a sense of security from their early life that predates the linguistic/verbal phase). Instead noticing how, beyond words, patients seem to change through what he calls "atmosphere," he has explored both verbal and non-verbal techniques in traditional and folk medicine, qi-philosophy, and martial arts, adopting and devising them to create a nurturing therapeutic space. He alternately induces regression in a "holding" environment and promotes insight through verbal reframing of a patient's problem (Kandabashi 2004). What is most controversial about Kandabashi's approach is the way in which he has invented and devised wide ranging therapeutic techniques, far beyond the reach of evidence-based medicine. He has encouraged patients to tap their fingers on medication to find what feels "right," and to lie down, pretend to be dead in order to experience quasi death and rebirth. He has promoted various deep breathing techniques as well as exercises using a "balance ball" (particularly for wrist cutters) in order to strengthen their inner trunk muscle – and, in turn, their core sense of the self. Having encountered so many patients who have severely suffered from the side effects of antipsychotics, Kandabashi prefers using traditional herbal medicine, regarding the brain as part of the whole body and teaching patients how to give them rest and to take better care of them (Kandabashi 1990 1999). Thus, while he is self-admittedly occultish, he is nonetheless in line with early pioneers of Japanese (psycho)therapy from the 1920s and 1930s, some practitioners of which were prominent doctors experimenting with deep breathing and other bodily approaches to neurasthenia (Wu 2016). In Freudian psychoanalysis, the body is regarded as primordial, something the rational mind can decode, revealing its truth and ultimately leading to liberation. From this perspective, Asians were depicted as primitive and preverbal "somatizers," contrasted with rational, intellectual, and more civilized "psychologizers" of the West (also for critique, see Kirmayer et al. 1998). More recently, however, a surprising reversal has occurred with the rise of mindfulness and other forms of breathing and meditation therapies, where the "Eastern" approach of achieving a balance of the mind through the body has gained credibility, dissolving former boundaries between the East and the West. In a similar vein, Kandabashi's translation of psychotherapy, which taps into the traditional philosophies, brings an understanding of the body as a rich source of profound wisdom and locus of agency.

How are these ideas put into practice? Thinking seriously about the harm psychiatry can do to patients

How do these ideas resonate with more general psychiatric practices, and in what ways do Japanese psychiatrists learn to be psychotherapeutic? In sharp contrast to the United States, where psychotherapy is required as part of official psychiatric training (Luhrmann 2000), in Japan, its training in medical schools is often limited to lectures, and the topic is far from systematically treated. Even in the university hospital where I did my fieldwork, which did offer a range of opportunities for studying psychotherapeutic approaches, doctors clearly gave priority to treating people with psychoses and prescribing antipsychotic medications, regarding the biomedical aspects of severe distress to be their primary responsibility. They operated largely on a medical model in order to quickly discern those who needed immediate psychiatric intervention and those who were more "neurotic," whom they felt might be better not to be "psychiatrized." Most patients did recover by medication and rest, along with what psychiatrists call "mini-psychotherapy," consisting of supportive listening and practical guidance that does not aim at inducing insight. As doctors explained, it was important for them to leave illness as something alien, not to be easily integrated with the self, in order to protect a patient's own sense of a healthy self. In hundreds of clinical cases I observed, psychiatrists would occasionally discuss among themselves psychoanalytic themes that emerge from patients' life histories and their current narratives, but such observations were often left for their own clinical insight and were not necessarily shared with patients or explicitly used in therapeutic processes.

There were a few exceptions, however, as with a case of a young salaryman who apparently became depressed from work stress and overwork (which is the prototype of depression in Japan: Kitanaka 2012). What made him unusual was that he kept posing existential questions about the meaning of his life, with which a young, psychotherapeutically minded doctor in training devotedly engaged. After what seemed like a steady recovery that brought the patient many insights, his symptoms began to worsen as his discharge date approached, as he became more aggressive and confrontational both in individual and group therapy settings. His discharge conference became a site of soul-searching for the doctors. While some residents suggested that he had borderline personality disorder, the professor immediately cautioned them against carelessly using a patient-blaming label and reminded them that the patient showed every sign of typical depression, explaining that the depressed often have deep-seated conflicts – underneath the seemingly normative, even ideal, hard-working, and caring personality – which could easily surface if not treated carefully. They talked about how threatening it was for this patient to confront his first major failure in life and how betrayed he must have felt upon realizing that doctors do not have the ultimate answer. While this case was highly unusual, residents in training were often warned to be wary of "magical and perverted thinking" that somehow they might change people. They would compare psychoanalytically oriented psychotherapy to surgery that should not be carelessly and casually experimented with: patients' searches for meaning can too often end up as a means of self-expression, producing a psychiatric patient identity and prolonging their ailment. It was thus safer to "provide a generic story" about depression, that it was a product of overwork that can be cured by rest. Doctors welcomed and cherished psychological insights that came to patients in the course of recovery, but they also knew how difficult it was for patients to confront their deeper problems once more superficial immediate problems were resolved.

In place of the psychological, psychiatrists went out of their way to offer both somatic and social interventions. Just as Nakai and Kandabashi emphasize the importance of somatic reflexivity, hospitalization was set up to allow patients to cultivate bodily sensibilities. Doctors talked about how patients tend to be filled with anxiety and emotions, so preoccupied with what is going on inside the mind that they tend to forget about and are alienated from their body. As the body is something concrete, graspable, and mutually observable, doctors felt it was useful to call attention to bodily changes as a way of making patients aware of their recovery and creating therapeutic alliance. Drawing on Nakai, they would talk about three kinds of fatigue: qi fatigue, which comes from the stress of human relations and thus is the hardest to deal with; brain fatigue, which can be healed through nature walks; and bodily fatigue, the easiest to deal with, as it can be cured simply by rest (Nakai 1982a:150). Outpatient consultation was set up to draw patients' awarenesses away from their psychological torments and instead nurture a holistic understanding of their own body, an insight that hundreds of patients I saw in case conferences and in my interviews seemed to genuinely appreciate. The overall message here was the power of body over mind and the transient and ephemeral nature of the psychological. To facilitate recovery, doctors also went out of their way to improve the environment to which patients would return, taking up the kind of tasks done by social workers in the United States. Doctors would call and invite to hospitals not just patients' families but also their company bosses to help them prepare more hospitable environments, advising them about the nature of a patient's illness, personality, work style, and prospects for recovery. It is only through such social intervention that they felt that psychological insights could be nurtured. This also reflects Japanese psychotherapists' awareness of the contradictory nature of psychological intervention that too often seems to them to go against the medical doctrine of "do no harm" (Kitanaka 2012).

Importantly, Japanese psychiatrists' caution against insight-inducing psychotherapeutic intervention is situated within their historical sensibility from more than a half century of failed therapeutic experiments. Nakai and Kandabashi came out of the vehement antipsychiatry movement, when psychiatrists were torn between astute self-criticism and the reality of continued practice of asylum psychiatry. In fact, Japan has infamously maintained the highest rates and lengths of psychiatric hospitalization in the world (the system little changed even after a decades-long antipsychiatry movement because of the strong lobbying force of private mental hospitals that dominate the field). In this context, psychotherapy developed as a tool for treating mainly schizophrenia in a preexisting hierarchical structure of the doctor–patient relationship characterized by strong paternalism. On the one hand, such an approach helped cultivate minute observational skills oriented to pathology and exploration of how best to protect fragile patients from the threat of ego diffusion and collapse, utilizing biomedical paternalism to therapeutic effect. This has also drawn on traditional philosophies about the intricate relationships between body and mind and the importance of patients' natural healing power towards recovery. On the other hand, because it was mainly presented as a set of bedside manners to be adopted and practiced by conscientious doctors, and not necessarily something for which doctors would have to go through rigorous training, the boundary of what is "psychotherapeutic" has remained ambiguous. In fact, "psychotherapeutic" has sometimes been equated with verbal encounters belonging to the more dominant German phenomenological and psychopathological traditions. Within this paradigm, the doctor remains the knower, the scientist, who coolly observes the patient. Such an approach assumes that pathology lies within the patient, and "talk" is used to reveal their underlying pathology in the absence of objective diagnostic tools for psychiatry (such as X-ray in other fields). Unfortunately, such "talking," where patients were made to discuss the minute details of their life and psychotic experiences, were at times misleadingly labeled as "psychotherapeutic," with little understanding of therapeutic contract, alliance, and/or patient autonomy that psychotherapy would entail. Some psychotherapists I met in the 2000s talked about having encountered tragic cases where patients who had been in an extended therapeutic relationship with a psychopathologically oriented doctor were "emptied out" of their inner world and seemingly cemented in their pathological experience.

In addition, given the near absence of systematic psychotherapeutic training in Japanese medical schools, doctors, even psychotherapeutically oriented ones, have not received rigorous supervision that would help instill in them critical self-reflexivity. Tanya Luhrmann, in her brilliant ethnography on the socialization of psychiatrists in the United States, discusses the contrasting "arrows of blame" that coexist in psychiatric training, arguing that while biological psychiatrists are taught how patients can harm them, psychotherapists learn how they can harm patients. She describes how residents in psychotherapy, through intensive sessions with borderline personality disorder patients, come to realize the extent to which the slightest gestures, facial expressions, and well-intended words can unwittingly hurt others. It is only through such critical and agonizing sessions that doctors come to acquire a true sense of empathy (Luhrmann 2000). In Japan, where there are so few places that offer such training for doctors, it is not surprising that clinical psychologists – who are increasingly going through such training and working in places like hospitals, clinics, and schools – are frustrated. Some psychologists I interviewed told me what little idea so-called psychotherapeutically oriented doctors seem to have of psychotherapy. They joke about doctors supposedly providing cognitive behavioral therapy instead giving a kind of "moral therapy," saying such outrageous things as "Try not to worry," without realizing that the reason the patient came to see them in the first place is because they do not know how not to worry. In open supervision at a psychiatric conference, Kandabashi gently walked a young doctor through a process of how to be more reflexive in his own words and actions. He did this without directly criticizing what seemed obvious to some in the audience: that the young doctor was, with all his sincerity and genuine commitment, little aware of his own countertransference and seemed to be acting out by prescribing more pills as an expression of his own aggression and frustration. Ironically, then, clinical psychologists in Japan often praise psychopharmaceutically oriented doctors for their lack of excessive/intrusive intervention and their modesty in knowing the limits of their own therapeutic power. Doctors who follow Nakai's model of psychotherapy on a superficial level may be able to operate largely within a medical model, as Nakai himself refrains from discussing his own feelings or patients' narratives in depth. Psychotherapy, understood as a set of bedside manners, becomes something safely applied to a biomedical setting and continues to dismiss psychoanalysis for its insistence on the irrational, emotional, and ambiguous, while aestheticizing its opposites – the rational, objective, and precision-seeking style of thinking (Shirahase 1997:415). As the economic environment of Japanese medicine changes, even Nakai's more medical model of psychotherapy – which prioritizes a patient's sense of security and promotes an untiring wait for "natural" recovery – may no longer be sustainable, as it is seen to create discharge delays. Indeed, with the accelerated pace and demand for recovery, the kind of clinical wisdom that Nakai and Kandabashi have preached may be barely thriving in doctors' consciences.

More recently, however, there have been multiple and creative attempts by Japanese psychotherapists to go beyond their limits, most notably a national movement that seeks to integrate "Open Dialogue," imported from Finland, into their practices. Prominent psychotherapist Tamaki Saito, a leading psychiatrist for treating *hikikomori* (social withdrawal, in which people lock themselves in their room for years, even decades, with little social interaction), has promoted Open Dialogue. Saito wonders if psychiatrists may have been led astray for over a century by Freud's greatest mistake, that in-depth dialogues between therapist and client in an isolated, closed room setting would somehow solve problems. Saito now argues that group settings in which people including the patient, family, therapists, and anyone else who cares for the patient gather to share feelings and thoughts openly, are so much gentler, fairer, and therapeutic for all involved. This would significantly reduce the weight of psychiatrists' words on a patient, who then begins to feel empowered and in control of the situation (Saito 2015b). This evokes the therapeutic principle of Kandabashi, who has sought to keep the highly "artificial" encounters of psychotherapy "shallow, narrow, short, and light" (Kandabashi 1990:41). Such attempts from psychiatrists also reflect the growing demand from patients to go beyond the traditional doctor–patient relationship, such as a rising user-activism in Japan called the "*tojisha kenkyu* movement." Its epicenter is a patient organization called Bethel that has done much to destigmatize mental illness by holding annual "delusion and hallucination contests" open to the public, where the person with the most hilarious delusion wins the prize. Those involved in Bethel have open meetings where they "study" and "research" their own psychoses, dissecting patterns and analyzing best intervention mechanisms (Nakamura 2013; Ishihara 2015). If psychotherapy is about cultivating autonomy and a sense of self-control, then these new movements address the gap in the traditionally medically dominated debates about psychotherapy in Japan (Borovoy 2005). For the time being, clinicians are aware of potential local resistance and criticisms against psychological intrusion, as well as limited resources and funding for long-term intervention, and are carefully maneuvering the boundaries of what or who constitutes a legitimate object of psychological intervention. Sensitive to the past criticisms against and grave failures of psychiatric intervention, they may be able to go beyond these to construe a truly effective but also not-so-intrusive form of psychological intervention.

The psychiatrization of the lifecycle and psychotherapy for dementia

Since the turn of the twenty-first century, psychiatrists have been facing an entirely new population of people seeking psychotherapeutic care in Japan. What initially brought this turn was the rise of depression in Japan from the late 1990s, creating a novel psychological landscape in which a massive number of people who had never thought of themselves as depressed are now actively seeking psychiatric care; some are taking up psychotherapy as well. If the rise of depression in the United States brought the "death of Freud" and *neurobiologization* (and *psychopharmaceuticalization*) of mental disorders, the same trend in Japan, where neurobiology had long dominated and psychotherapy had little significance, may actually be bringing the opposite effect of *psychologization* (or at least *psychiatrization*) of everyday distress. What partly drives the popularization of psychiatric reflexivity is the fact that depression has come to be reconceptualized in this country as an illness of stress and overwork, and as such has rapidly become a concern in the workplace across the nation. After a series of successful litigations against corporations by families of deceased workers allegedly driven to depression and suicide from work stress, both the government and industries have begun to look into ways to monitor and intervene in stressed and mentally distressed workers. Their concerns are heightened particularly because companies can now be held liable for failing to foresee the risk of depression and suicide even when the worker him/herself is unaware of his/her depression. The government has installed a number of policy changes in labor law, including the 2015 implementation of so-called stress checks for mental health screening of workers nationwide. As these stress checks ask multiple and detailed questions not just about the stress of the workplace and the environment but also the individual workers' psychological health, people are becoming "aware" of their psychological states in a new light, potentially cultivating fertile ground for psychotherapeutic intervention. Indeed, as more and more people are realizing the limits of psychopharmaceutical intervention, stating how in the long term they have to confront the way they live and work, and as they seek help in the vast number of mental health clinics that have mushroomed in the 2000s, new spaces of psychological engagements that go clearly against the former interdiction of psychotherapy are opening up (Kitanaka 2015).

As detecting and preventing depression in young and middle-aged workers has become an urgent national imperative, there is also a concurrent move to screen and intervene in children with developmental disorders as well as among the elderly for signs of dementia. This has created what I call "the psychiatrization of lifecycle," where lay people are increasingly adopting psychiatric/psychological language to reflect upon their senses of healthy selves at certain junctures in their lives. I am particularly interested in the fact that, just as Nakai and Kandabashi discussed decades ago, mental health in old age in particular has become everyone's concern in a society that is currently leading the world for its status as the "super aging society." People with (the risk and fear of) dementia have suddenly emerged as a potential set of clientele for psychotherapy. Nakai discussed in 1982 that the then-current state of psychopathological knowledge about dementia was so impoverished (he called it a "dark continent") that it resembled the manners in which schizophrenia used to be talked about as a "brain disease" in psychiatry in the 1910s, with psychiatrists assuming that there was not much clinically interesting to be explored (Nakai 2011:184). The flourishing of psychopathological, phenomenological, and psychotherapeutic discussions on schizophrenia from the 1950s on has led to entirely different ways of looking at (and experiencing) schizophrenia and has led to novel approaches like Open Dialogue discussed earlier. While discussions about dementia today center on neurological findings and biomedical intervention, there is also increasing attention to people's subjectivity and affective experiences of dementia and how to intervene, psychotherapeutically, to help them cope with and engage in the process of gradual self-transformation as well as their fear of impending death. Yumiko Nagano, veteran psychotherapist, told me that doing psychotherapy with people in their sixties and beyond resembles in some ways psychotherapy with adolescents; members of both age groups struggle with the fact that their own senses of self (constantly shifting given their physiological changes) are not necessarily in accord with the way they are (or they would like or imagine to be) seen by others, creating discrepancies rife with tension and conflicts, while complicating issues about autonomy and dependency.

Dementia does pose unique problems for psychotherapists. Because of the degenerative, progressive character of the disease, it is difficult to set a therapeutic goal for recovery and closure. And, perhaps more importantly, the impediment dementia brings to one's memory and use of language poses serious challenges to a psychotherapy that relies heavily on the idea of the narrative self. Perhaps it is this ideal of the self as a narrative-based sense of coherence, which implies interiority, integrity, a depth in a person, that imposes unnecessary pressure on both those with dementia and those who care for them. The pervasive worries about memory, perhaps a contemporary form of obsession, strengthened by the rise of the vision of hyper cerebral, neurochemical selves (Rose 2007), may also contribute to the dread that people feel towards those who show serious signs of aging. If it is this historically specific construction of the self that is partly tormenting people with dementia, making them feel as if they are reducible to demented brains, then I wonder if the kinds of multiple approaches to psychotherapy that Japanese psychotherapists have long explored, and which continue to question and argue against the Freudian model of health and personhood, might not be helpful in creating novel ways for reimagining psychotherapy that goes well beyond words. It is perhaps through an engagement with this stage of the lifecycle that the Japanese "psychotherapeutic" insistence that there should be different ways of conceptualizing the self – that there should not be only one prioritizing rationality, autonomy, and boundedness but rather multiple ways of being that can be intersubjective, interdependent, fragmented, and unbounded – may be put to a test.

This work was supported by JSPS KAKENHI Grant Number JP16KT0123.

References

Araki, F. (1997) Kandabashi sensei ni tsuiteno renso (Association about Dr. Kandabashi). In Fukuoka kodo igaku kenkyujo, *Aru atsumari no kioku: Kandabashi Joji sensei kanreki kinenshu (Memory of a gathering: Collected essays for celebrating the 60th birthday of Dr. Kandabashi Joji)*. Fukuoka: Iryohojin uraume no sato kai. Pp. 1–8.

Borovoy, A. (2005) *The too-good wife: Alcohol, codependency, and the politics of nurturance in postwar Japan*. Berkeley: University of California Press.

Borovoy, A. (forthcoming) *Japan in American social thought: Experiments in modernity, community, and cultural relativism*. Princeton, NJ: Princeton University Press.

Corin, E. & G. Lauzon. (1992) Positive withdrawal and the quest for meaning: The reconstruction of experience among schizophrenics. *Psychiatry* 55(3): 266–278.

Doi, T. (1972) Bunretsubyō to himitsu (schizophrenia and secrets). In T. Doi (Ed.), *Bunretsubyō no seishinbyōri (The psychopathology of schizophrenia)*. Tokyo: Tokyo University Press. Pp. 1–18.

Doi, T. (1973) *The anatomy of dependence*. Tokyo; New York: Kodansha International.

Doi, T. (1990) The cultural assumptions of psychoanalysis. In J. W. Stigler, R. A. Shweder, G. H. Herdt & University of Chicago Committee on Human Development (Eds.), *Cultural psychology: Essays on comparative human development*. Cambridge; New York: Cambridge University Press.

Fujiyama, N. (2010) Seishin bunseki wa seishinka iryo ni totte donoyouna imi ga arunoka (What meaning does psychoanalysis have for psychiatric medicine?). In S. Kanba & M. Matsushita (Eds.), *Seishin igaku no shiso (Ideas in psychiatry)*. Tokyo: Nakayama Shoten. Pp. 175–190.

Fukuoka kodo igaku kenkyujo. (1997) *Aru atsumari no kioku: Kandabashi Joji sensei kanreki kinenshu (Memory of a gathering: Collected essays for celebrating the 60th birthday of Dr. Kandabashi Joji)*. Fukuoka: Iryohojin uraume no sato kai.

Fukuoka kodo igaku kenkyujo. (2007) *Hitotsu no ayumi: Kandabashi Joji sensei koki kinenshu (A path: Collected essays for celebrating the 70th birthday of Dr. Kandabashi Joji)*. Fukuoka: Iryohojin uraume no sato kai.

Harding, C. (2014) Japanese psychoanalysis and Buddhism: The making of a relationship. *History of Psychiatry* (June).

Hazuki, S. (2014) *Therapist: Silence in Psychotherapy*. Tokyo: Shinchosha.

Hirosawa, M. (2015) Togo shiccho kanja eno mensetsu ni nozomu shisei (Stance towards consultation with a schizophrenic patient). *Kokoro no kagaku (Human mind)* Special Issue: 81–84.

Ishihara, K. (2015) Learning from tojisha kenkyu: Mental health "patients" studying their difficulties with their peers. In T. Shakespeare (Ed.), *Disability research today: International perspectives*. London: Routledge. Pp. 27–42.

Kanba, S. (2014) Commentary on Kandabashi's Sokyokusei shogai no shindan to chiryo (Diagnosis and treatment for bipolar disorders). In S. Kanba et al. (Ed.), *Watashi no Rinsho Seishin Igaku: Kyudai Seishinka Kogiroku (My perspectives on clinical psychiatry: Lectures at Kyushu university psychiatric department)*. Osaka: Sogensha.

Kandabashi, J. (1984) *Seishinka shindan mensetsu no kotsu (Keys to psychiatric diagnostic interview)*. Tokyo: Iwasaki gakujutsu shuppansha.

Kandabashi, J. (1988) *Hasso no koseki (Trajectory of thoughts)*. Tokyo: Iwasaki gakujutsu shuppansha.

Kandabashi, J. (1988[1974]). Himitsu no yakuwari (the role of the "secret"). In *Hassō no kōseki (trajectory of thoughts)*. Tokyo: Iwasaki Gakujutsu Shuppansha.

Kandabashi, J. (1990) *Seishinryoho mensetsu no kotsu (Keys to psychotherapeutic interview)*. Tokyo: Iwasaki gakujutsu shuppansha.

Kandabashi, J. (1999) *Seishinka yojo no kotsu (keys to Psychiatric health)*. Tokyo: Iwasaki gakujutsu shuppansha.
Kandabashi, J. (2004) *Hasso no koseki II (Trajectory of thoughts II)*. Tokyo: Iwasaki gakujutsu shuppansha.
Kandabashi, J. (2011) *Waza wo hagukumu (Cultivating techniques)*. Tokyo: Nakayama shoten.
Kandabashi, J. (2013) *Igakubu kobi (Medical school lectures)*. Osaka: Sogensha.
Kandabashi, J. (2016) *Chiryo no tameno seishinbunseki noto (Psychoanalytic notes for treatment)*. Osaka: Sogensha.
Kirmayer, L., T. Dao, T. Hong & A. Smith. (1998) Somatization and psychologization: Understanding cultural idioms of distress. In S. O. Okpaku (Ed.), *Clinical methods in transcultural psychiatry*. Washington, DC: American Psychiatric Press.
Kitanaka, J. (2003) Jungians and the rise of psychotherapy in Japan: A brief historical note. *Transcultural Psychiatry* 40(2) (June): 239–247.
Kitanaka, J. (2012) *Depression in Japan: Psychiatric cures for a society in distress*. Princeton, NJ: Princeton University Press.
Kitanaka, J. (2015) The rebirth of secrets and the new care of the self in depressed Japan. *Current Anthropology* 56(12): S251–S262.
Kleinman, A. (1991) *Rethinking psychiatry: From cultural category to personal experience*. New York: Free Press.
Kuroki, T. (2015) Seishinka yakubutsu ryoho no saho (Methods of psychiatric pharmaceuticology). *Kokoro no kagaku (Human Mind)* Special Issue: 76–80.
Luhrmann, T. M. (2000) *Of two minds: The growing disorder in American psychiatry*. New York: Knopf.
Mauss, M. (1985) A category of the human mind. In M. Carrithers, S. Collins & S. Lukes (Eds.), *The category of the person: Anthropology, philosophy, history*. Cambridge: Cambridge University Press. Pp. 1–25.
Morita, S. (1998) *Morita therapy and the true nature of anxiety-based disorders* (Eds.), Kondo, A. & LeVine, P. New York: State University of New York Press.
Mouer, R. & Y. Sugimoto. (1986) *Images of Japanese society: A study in the social construction of reality*. London; New York: Kegan Paul International.
Murase, K. & S. Aoki. (2014) *Shinri ryoho no kihon: Nichijo rinsho no tame no teigen (Foundations of psychotherapy: Proposals for everyday clinical practice)*. Tokyo: Kongo shuppan.
Nakai, H. (1976) Saiken no rinri to shite no kinben to kufu (Diligence and innovation as an ethic of reconstruction). In Y. Kasahara (Ed.), *Sōutsubyō no Seishinbyōri I (Psychopathology of Manic Depression)*. Tokyo: Kōbundō.
Nakai, H. (1979) Kimyona shizukesa to zawameki to hishimeki (Strange tranquility, rumble of voices and crammers). In H. Nakai (Ed.), *Bunretsubyo no seishinbyori vol. 8 (Psychopathology of schizophrenia, vol. 8)*. Tokyo: Tokyo University Press.
Nakai, H. (1982a) *Seishinka chiryo no oboegaki (Memorandum for psychiatric treatment)*. Tokyo: Nihon hyoronsha.
Nakai, H. (1982b) *Bunretsubyo to jinrui (Schizophrenia and human species)*. Tokyo: Tokyo University Press.
Nakai, H. (2010) *Nihon no isha (Doctors in Japan)*. Tokyo: Nihon hyoronsha.
Nakai, H. (2011) *Tsunagari no seishinbyori (Psychopathology of connection)*. Tokyo: Chikuma Shobo.
Nakai, H. et al. (1983) *Chiryō to Bunka (Therapy and culture)*. Vol. 8. Iwanami Koza: Seishin No Kagaku (Science of the Mind). Tokyo: Iwanami Shoten.
Nakamura, K. (2013) *A disability of the soul: An ethnography of schizophrenia and mental illness in contemporary Japan*. Ithaca, NY: Cornell University Press.

Okonogi, K. (1982) *Nihonjin no ajase konpurekkusu (Japanese Ajase complex)*. Tokyo: Chuo koronsha.

Okubo, K. (2015) Nakai sensei no rinsho saho (Clinical methods of Dr. Nakai). *Kokoro no kagaku (Human Mind)* Special Issue: 72–75.

Rose, N. (2007) *The politics of life itself: Biomedicine, power, and subjectivity in the twenty-first century*. Princeton, NJ: Princeton University Press.

Saio, T. (2011) *Seishinkai: Kakusareta Shinjitu (Psychiatrists: Hidden truths)*. Tokyo: Toyokeizaishinposha.

Saito, T. (2015a) Joshiki to shite no "Komoji no seishinryoho" (Small-letter "psychotherapy" as a commonsense). *Kokoro no kagaku (Human Mind)* Special Issue: 68–71.

Saito, T. (2015b) *Opun daiarogu to wa nanika (What is open dialogue?)*. Tokyo: Igaku Shoin.

Shirahase, J. (1997) Seishin ryoho/seishin bunseki teki seishin ryoho (Psychotherapy/psychoanalytic psychotherapy). In M. Matsushita & E. Kishimoto (Eds.), *Kanjo shogai: Kiso to rinsho (Affective disorders: Foundations and clinical practice)*. Tokyo: Asakura Shoten. (CHECK). Uchimura, Y. (1954) Nihon seishin igaku no kako to shōrai (Past and future of Japanese psychiatry). *Seishin Shinkeigaku Zasshi (Journal of Psychiatry and Neurology)* 55(7).

Wu, Y. (2016) Straighten the back to sit: Belly-cultivation techniques as "modern health methods" in Japan, 1900–1945. *Culture, Medicine and Psychiatry* 40(3): 450–474.

3

RELATING WITH OR WITHOUT CULTURE

Inga-Britt Krause

Introduction

When I, twenty-five years or so ago, first trained in systemic psychotherapy, also sometimes referred to as family therapy, I was surprised to discover several publications by Gregory Bateson which had not played any significant role in my life as a social anthropologist. These were collected in the volume entitled *Steps to an Ecology of Mind* (Bateson, 1972b) and also in the book *Mind and Nature* (Bateson, 1979). I knew and had been intrigued by Bateson's maverick work in social anthropology (Ingold, 1986; Marcus, 1985) and his ethnographic study *Naven. The Culture of the Iatmul People of New Guinea as Revealed Through a Study of the 'Naven' Ceremonial* (Bateson, 1958). My surprise and puzzlement were on two counts. First, because Bateson was and still is considered a founding figure in cybernetics and later systemic psychotherapy – the latter not really emerging as a psychotherapy approach until some time after the Macy conferences in the 1940s – and yet as a social anthropologist I knew nothing and had heard nothing about this. Second, because hardly anyone in the systemic psychotherapy field at the time of my training had read or even referred to *Naven* (1958). Nor were the more ethnographic papers in *Steps to an Ecology of Mind* (Bateson, 1972b) referred to or studied. Systemic psychotherapy trainees and students would read and almost as dogma refer to papers such as "Toward a Theory of Schizophrenia" (1956) co-authored by Bateson with psychiatrists (Bateson, Jackson, Hayley, & Weakland, 1956), "Double Bind" (1972b) and "The Cybernetic of 'Self': A Theory of Alcoholism" (1971). However, reading "Style, Grace, and Information in Primitive Art" (1972a) or "Culture Contact and Schismogenesis" (1935) or "Bali: The Value System of a Steady State" (1949) was not encouraged, despite these papers sitting side by side with the psychiatric ones in the same volume. Bateson had developed the idea of schismogenesis – which, as I shall describe, became fundamental to systemic thinking about relationships – in the first 1939 edition of the book *Naven*, but references to this idea, while frequently made in systemic psychotherapy/family therapy, were always to the psychiatric papers in *Steps*.

I do not think that this emphasis reflected an idea that the two fields, anthropology and psychiatry/systemic psychotherapy, were irrelevant to each other. Rather, the split expressed in the selective emphasis on reading material articulated a tension or a conflict between Bateson's ethnographic work and the clinical work or encounter in the therapy room as practised and conceptualised at the end of the 1980s in systemic psychotherapy and still with us today. Ethnographic details were considered as more or less irrelevant and certainly not of concern for practising psychotherapists (I remember well my astonishment and irritation when one of my teachers, who I respected then as I do now, told me that two to three minutes into a family therapy session I would be able to understand what is going on). The issue hinged on 'culture' (Krause, 2007), and as I later learnt, there had been an actual rift between Bateson and his closest colleagues, precisely about how to include 'culture' in a theory of communication (Harries-Jones, 1995; Krause, 2007). The communications project on which Bateson had been working with his psychiatric colleagues in Palo Alto and which also became one foundation for the discipline of systemic psychotherapy took the discipline in a behavioural direction with echoes of the structural functionalism of Talcott Parsons and Radcliffe-Brown; questions about power, gender and cultural differences did not generally enter thinking and/or practice in systemic psychotherapy till about the time when I began my training at the end of the 1980s, this being in tune with the general shift following the crisis in representation prevailing in the social sciences at that time. In systemic psychotherapy, we speak about the shift from 'first order', referring to the psychotherapist considering herself 'outside' the system of the family, and to different degrees 'directing' change to 'second order', in which the therapist considers herself as a participant in 'the system/family'; this is accompanied by the assumption that while she may be able to facilitate different conversations by being in some way an expert conversationalist (Anderson and Goolishan, 1988), she cannot know and therefore direct the system or the participants in it in any particular direction. This is a dominant stance in the discipline in the UK currently.

What, then, can we learn about 'culture' from the tensions and dilemmas, intersections and divergences of anthropology and psychotherapy? And what might this tell us about method and about the interface between ethnography as a method of enquiry and systemic psychotherapy enquiry in practice? And how do these two questions relate to each other in the two disciplines? In contrast to other chapters in this volume, I want to argue that not only does anthropology have much to offer systemic psychotherapists, but systemic psychotherapy can also assist anthropologists and ethnographers with how to enquire and how to think about the relationships between themselves and their interlocutors.

Bateson, anthropology and the systemic psychotherapist

As I indicated, the collaboration between Bateson and psychiatry really took off after Bateson discovered cybernetics (Harries-Jones, 1995), and an important idea in the discipline became that of 'feed-back' or 'self-correction', offering an explanation of why interaction and communication in relationships between persons can be seen to make up patterns, which are (more or less) repeated over time. In families seen in psychiatric clinics, such patterns are sometimes stuck and inflexible, leading to serious symptoms and unhappiness. However, the inspiration of this idea actually derived from Bateson's ethnographic work on the *naven*[1] ritual before his involvement with cybernetics. In this ritual, a mother's brother marked his sister's son achieving adult status by dressing up in decrepit women's clothes, chasing the young man and, when catching him, rubbing his buttocks against the young man's thigh in a gesture with sexual connotations (a gesture called *nggariik*; (Silverman, 2001)). The sister's son then was obliged to present something to his mother's brother in return. There were echoes of this transvestite behaviour in other relationships, too, for example involving a girl and a father's sister. The ritual included inversions of dominant and expected gender roles and emotional outlooks in that women dressed up as men and men as women each simulated and acquired some kind of experience of the behaviour and emotional outlook of the other gender, of being the other. From these observations, Bateson developed the notion of 'schismogenesis', referring to the process in which contrasting, symmetrical or complementary emotional outlooks, behaviours or communications are produced and maintained by their own dynamic. Schismogenesis captures how persons react to one another, how these accumulated and repeated reactions constitute social patterns and how such social patterns may exist and be maintained, restrained or changed as a result of both their own dynamic and the dynamic of other social patterns with which they come into contact. This work, then, was an attempt at the beginnings of a generic theory of relationships.

From time to time in my readings while a student of anthropology, and later when interested in the relationship between anthropology and psychotherapy, I have come across anthropologists who have written about schismogenesis and its significance for how we might think about emotional and psychological dispositions in social relationships while still keeping in mind the influence of wider social contexts. Two such significant contributions are those of Nuckolls (Nuckolls, 1996) and Silverman (Silverman, 2001). While Nuckolls pointed to references which Bateson himself (somewhat ambivalently) made to Freud and draws a parallel between the dialectic seen by Freud to operate in the mind and in the unconscious of individuals to that seen by Bateson to operate in social interaction through ritual, the analysis by Silverman picked up on Bateson's point about *naven* achieving psychological integration for individual persons and cast his analysis in terms of unconscious desire, the envy men feel for women (mothers) and the ambivalent place of masculinity in this society. Neither of these two writers locate their enquiry in the area of the minutiae of actual communications and interactions between persons outside the *naven* ritual and do not seem to be aware of (at least they do not refer to) the importance of Bateson's ideas for systemic psychotherapy.

Recently, however, Ingold, who is no stranger to the work of Bateson, has described anthropology as a 'discipline of correspondence' (Ingold, 2017, p. 24), in terms which to my mind point to some resonance between anthropology and systemic psychotherapy. Ingold begins with the image of 'taking another by the hand' and elaborates this into 'joining with' and Dewey's notion of "having things in common being not a prerequisite but an outcome of communication" (Dewey, 1966:4, quoted in Ingold, 2017, p. 14). Ingold explains,

> to have in common is not to look inside ourselves, to regress to a set of baseline attributes with which we are similarly endowed from the start, but to reach out to others who are – at least initially – different from us.
>
> *(Ingold, 2017, pp. 14–15)*

In language which could have been used to describe schismogenesis, Ingold refers to *interstitial differentiation* as "the way in which difference continually arises from within the midst of joining *with*, in the ongoing sympathy of going along together" (Ingold, 2017, p. 13) and feedback as the "attentional movement in which the movement resonates with the things to which it attends" (p. 18). The theory of correspondence is a premise for getting inside relationships, in the sense that one can be inside the in-between. It is not *of*-ness (making an object of that to which one attends), but *with*-ness, which "brings it alongside as a fellow traveller" (p. 24).

Ingold's discipline of correspondence articulates the very principle upon which the process of being an anthropologist, that is to say both a participant and an observer, is based and as such is a condition for the carrying out of ethnography. Much of what Ingold says also resonates with contemporary systemic psychotherapy, in which the discipline of correspondence can be said to be a fundamental principle articulating both a stance (of joining with) and an emphasis on technique. Indeed, a similar idea has been articulated by Shotter, whose writings are influential in contemporary systemic psychotherapy (Shotter, 2010). I shall return to what systemic psychotherapists can learn from anthropologists below, but for now I want to suggest that anthropologists can learn from systemic psychotherapy clinical practice how to further their own skills in developing the discipline of correspondence from which their ethnographic understanding inevitably emerges. In what follows I use a case example to show how I and a colleague worked with a mother and her son, aiming to stay alongside both as well as to get inside the differences in the relationship between them.

Family or systemic psychotherapy

Many of the most influential family therapists who were pioneers in the discipline of systemic psychotherapy were themselves trained psychoanalysts and made use of this prior training and experience in their work with families, without ever directly writing about this. They found working with individuals by themselves limiting and instead began to work with families in the consulting room. In brief, the idea was that communication and behaviour in families contribute to and in some instances maintain the symptoms experienced by individual members. By aiming to help family members know new things about each other or understand each other in new ways, and by working with them on how to communicate differently and have different conversations, the problem, for which they have sought help, may become more bearable and in some instances disappear. There are overtones of social functionalism (Bateson's supervisor in social anthropology at Cambridge was Radcliffe-Brown (Harries-Jones, 1995)), and the view from the therapy room, or rather from the observation room (systemic psychotherapists are well known for working with one-way-mirrors through which supervision is live and members of a whole team actively participate in the therapy process), generally was one of the 'here and now'. If, in the therapy room, families could be helped to experience something which was different from the usual pattern, this might encourage a change, and a new pattern might give rise to new communications and different ways of relating at home. Initially this also meant that while therapists might have been interested in the history and development of individual persons in relationships with others and in the history of symptoms, with few exceptions (for example, Boyd-Franklin, 1989; Falicov, 1995; Minuchin et al., 1967) the wider social and political history and the social ideologies and processes, which were the contexts for the lives of persons and families, were not of primary interest. This had normative implications, and alternative cultural outlooks and theories at first rarely entered the therapists' thinking, except in those instances, which were few and far between, when the therapist him (therapists were mostly male) or herself came from backgrounds other than white and Euro-American. These outlooks have shifted somewhat since the 1980s, so that for example the social context may be thought to be more important, while at the same time it has also become more common for systemic psychotherapists to work with individuals using a systemic perspective. This shift has been accompanied by an increasing dominance of social constructionist and narrative approaches and has had implications for the life of the 'culture concept' in the discipline.

The manner in which the systemic psychotherapist enquires is thus aimed at opening up information, new ideas, thoughts and experiences for the psychotherapist, but importantly also for families and family members. In the epistemology of cybernetics, which Bateson came to see as a model for social or family systems (Krause, 2002), he stated this in a well-known quote that has become iconic for the discipline,

> A 'bit' of information is definable as a difference which makes a difference. Such a difference, as it travels and undergoes successive transformation in a circuit, is an elementary idea. But most relevant in the present context, we know that no part of such an internally interactive system can have

> unilateral control over the remainder or over any other part. The mental characteristics are inherent or immanent in the ensemble as a *whole*.
>
> *(Bateson, 1972b, p. 315, italics in the text)*

The therapist and the family in their encounter in the therapy room aim to discover 'a difference which makes a difference', and towards this end the systemic psychotherapist has a repertoire of techniques, which may have been picked up by, but are not characteristic of, other therapeutic approaches. Some of these are associated with earlier schools of family therapy, such as Milan and structural family therapy, while others have been added more recently; all are now taught as tools of therapeutic practice on systemic psychotherapy programmes in the UK. These include genograms, circular questions, reflecting statements, systemic summaries, interventive statements, reflexivity, relational reflexivity, hypothesising, externalising and the use of ideas such as circularity, neutrality and positive connotation. Some of these techniques are used in the extract from a therapy session below.

This extract is from a session with a family of a mixed-race mother (F) aged about 40, of Afro-Caribbean background, and her two mixed-race children, M, who is 13, and E, who is 10 and does not currently take part in the sessions. The mother has a female partner and has not lived with the children's father since M was very small, at which point F moved out following a series of incidents of abuse and controlling behaviour by the father. F also suffered sexual abuse as a child and has a difficult relationship to her own mother. I (B), a white Danish middle-aged woman, and my colleague (A), a younger black male trainee child psychotherapist of Ghanaian descent, have been working with the family for a few months. A worked with M prior to my involvement, providing child psychotherapy sessions. However, M did not engage and found it extremely hard to separate from his mother in the waiting room before each session. It was therefore decided that family therapy might help work these issues through and that M would eventually go back to having his own individual psychotherapy with A as his psychotherapist. This background to the work presents a number of issues, which I note in passing. Firstly, I and my colleague have different histories with the family. Secondly, we are of different degrees of experience and seniority as well as trained in different modalities of psychotherapy, I in systemic psychotherapy and my colleague in Kleinian child psychoanalytic psychotherapy. Generally, we are both sympathetic to the approach of the other, but there are times when we struggle to find coherence between the two approaches. The sequence quoted here is not one of these. Finally, we are from different social backgrounds and have different skin colour. The details below derive from a therapy session, which is part of a sequence of sessions in which we are working to understand M's and F' s relationship, which at times is volatile with M physically hurting his mother. The sequence is transcribed verbatim from a video recording, to which the family have given consent. This is standard practice in systemic psychotherapy, especially if a one-way mirror is not available. It allows the therapists to review their work as well as to share the recording with the family. I have just asked M what he has been doing during the recent Easter break.

M: Friends came over – we had a sleep over . . .
B: What has mum been doing . . .?
M: I do not really know – I was pretty much out . . .except for night time when I came back . . .
A: What were you doing out . . .?
M: . . . riding my bike . . .
B: at those times does that mean you argue more or less in the house?
M: Well I do not know – it will probably be less . . . because I might be having arguments when I stay in, but more . . . because at nighttimes we have arguments . . .
B: Hm . . .
B: About going to bed and stuff? . . . have they been worse than normal or is it pretty normal that children have arguments in the holidays?
M: It was a bit bad recently, but it was not like . . . but it is much better than it used to be . . .
B: Do you imagine mum agrees with you . . .?
M: I do not know . . .
B: What do you imagine?
M: I do not know . . . she probably thinks the same . . .
F: . . . . . probably thinks the same as what you think?
B: Sometimes we might imagine that mums think 'no, that is not true' . . . but you think that she thinks it is a fair assessment?
M: yes . . .
B: Shall we ask her?
M: Yeah . . .
B: (to F) Is it?
F: It is a very fair assessment . . . M has been taking his medication now for two weeks . . . and I think we are both agreed that this is definitely helping.

I am asking a series of circular questions, that is to say questions to one person about the other or about others. These questions are aimed at enquiring into how a person thinks another person sees or understands him or her and in this way is directly aimed at the in-between of their relationship. For example, M does not know what his mother has been doing while he has been out, whereas another child might have a good idea or might have been told or be preoccupied by this. Nor is M sure that his mother sees their arguments in the same way as he does. However, rather than this being a sign that M and his mother have actually been getting on better, we also hear that M thinks that they have had fewer arguments because they have not been together, not really because they have actually been getting on better or because he expected them to get on better. On the other hand, 'being out riding his bike' may be a way of staying safe from the arguments, which have been happening at night. We find out that these arguments are less than they used to be and, finally and importantly, that they agree on this last point. The way in which the conversation unfolded was tentative and I felt I was walking on eggshells when I asked the first series of circular questions. It also seemed that F did not want to stay with the quality of their relationship, so although she said she agreed with M, she quickly shifted the emphasis and attributed the 'slight' improvement to the ADHD medication. I felt that there could not be space for hope that something could be better. This is despite the fact that I stated what we might call a hypothesis, which was also an invitation to have a disagreement, when I said that parents and children do not always agree and that this would be normal. A and I discussed afterwards whether it is simply impossible for F and M to have a small disagreement that can be worked through without it developing into a big argument. We are receiving information about connectedness in their relationship but also about disconnection. Without the former it would be difficult to work therapeutically with the latter idea, that M is better only because he is taking medication. So, aiming to understand how the ADHD medication enters into their relationship, I ask two additional circular questions along the same lines:

B: How do you know when the medication is working because most children and parents we know argue about stuff? How do you know when the medication is working in a good way or not in a good way?

And

B: Do you think that mum has tried harder to get on or is it all up to what you have done?

Later on in the session, we are turning our attention in another direction, which my colleague and I had already decided would be important. M has just tied his mother's shoelaces from different shoes together and he has lost the thread of our conversation. I have asked whether F minds M doing this and she said that compared to all the things he might do, this is minor and not worth having an issue with. We wonder whether the intensity of the topic is too much.

M: Everything here has to be a big question . . . .

B: I am wondering whether it is hard to talk, especially about serious things . . . but this reminds me that there was something which A and I wanted to ask . . . . what do you think about coming here? About what we do here?

F: M was clear that he did not want to talk today . . . he did not want to come . . . . .

B: . . . . . . So you did not want to come, but you came anyway?

M: She would not let me go out if I did not come. I did not want to come here in the holidays . . . . .

B: Yes, a lot of children do not want to come in the holidays . . . we understand that . . . . but you have been here before when it was no holidays . . . . so what do you think about coming here those other times?

M: I don't know. Mummy thinks it is good . . . .

Here my colleague and I have decided to address coming to therapy and the way this is experienced as a comment on the process of the therapy. We are enquiring about not what has happened and how this can be understood (content) but about what is happening (process) here between us. M is becoming increasingly restless, kicking his mother's foot, trying her reflexes (knee) and tying her shoelaces together. This feels as if he wants to distract us, but it also feels aggressive and we wondered later whether he is getting back at his mother for bringing him to the therapy. Prompted by M saying "everything has to be such a big question", we ask a question which aims at what systemic psychotherapists refer to as relational reflexivity, i.e. what do M and F think about us and what we are doing here.

Still later in the session the following exchange takes place, which begins with a question referring to talking about talking.

B: Do you know why A and I want you to come here to therapy?

M: I do not know . . . . (takes a long time) . . . . . . because I had a bit of trouble when I was younger and because I have ADHD . . . .

A: Do you ever imagine what is going to happen in the future. Do you imagine how long you are going to come?

M: What . . . . .?

A: Do you ever imagine how long you are going to come time wise?

M: Mummy says we are going to therapy today . . . I do not think about how long it will last.

A: Do you ever imagine what might happen what it might feel like or what needs to change for me and B to say that you do not need to come anymore or for mummy to say there is no need to go to therapy anymore?

M: What that would feel like for me if I do not need to come any more? . . . . I don't know . . . kind of . . . what would have to happen for me to stop coming ? . . . I do not know . . . but if I did stop coming I do not think that I would be really upset. I do not really keep a record . . . . I do not really count the days . . . . . .

B: Hm. . I was thinking although that is a good question, we do not know when you do not need to come anymore . . . . . we do not know that yet and we might have to think about that sometime, but I was also thinking that the reason that we like you to come sometimes is that we also think that sometimes it is hard for children to get their point of view across . . . and maybe they do not even know their point of view till they kind of had an opportunity to think about this . . . so we know that children can be . . . .

M: (interrupting to F and squirming on his chair) what time is it?

F: It was a quarter to 11 . . . . .
B: Does that make sense?
M: I did not hear you . . . . (M is fiddling with his phone) . . . . .
B: Well if you were really cross with mum and you might not be able to say it except in this way that you have been saying it when you get very cross, it might be a way for you to say it here . . . .
F: Put your phone down M!. . . . .
B: Most children get cross with their parents . . . it would not be unusual . . . . . .
M: I do get cross with mum . . . .
F: Please put the phone down . . . .!
M: I can't see the time . . . . . .
F: You and I both know that is not true . . . so it is just rude, please put it down!
M: It is 10.48 . . . . you are lying . . . .
F: It was a quarter to 11 . . . when I looked at B's watch . . . . it is really rude to stay on your phone, please put it down . . . . . .
M: You are lying . . . . are you going to look like granny when you get older?
F: Am I going to look like granny when I am older . . . .!
M: Yes you look exactly like granny . . . . . .
F: I do not look exactly like granny, I am brown, she is white . . . . that is one difference . . . .
M: I still don't . . . . all my friends say that you are brown . . . .
F: I *am* brown . . . .
M: You are darker than . . . like . . . B . . . . .
B: So is granny white . . . . .?
F: Yes.
B: So what about M's dad?
F: he . . . is . . . .
M: Not as dark as me . . . .
F: How dark is daddy? Is he darker than you . . . is he darker than you?. . . . . . . probably
M: A tiny bit darker than E (M's younger brother).
F: What a bit darker than you. .?
M: E is brown and I am mixed race and . . . . he is more brown
B: Is that what you call yourself when you think about yourself . . . .?
M: Yes I don't think . . . . . I would not call myself black and I would not call, I would not call myself white either . . . .
F: Technically you are absolutely correct . . . you are mixed . . .
M: E is a bit darker . . . . . .
F: He is mixed race as well . . . .
B: So you would call me white?
M: yes
B: And what would you call A?
M: Black . . . .
F: We have had some developments recently . . . M wants to write to his dad . . . .

In this section, the conflict intensified, and it seemed to us that F was not sure what to do. She did not want to provoke M by stopping him tying her shoelaces together. However, it also became too much for her and she lashed out towards M about the phone. He then retaliated by referring to her likeness to her mother. At that point I remember thinking that M was provoking his mother by tying her shoelaces together so that she would not be able to walk and that this seemed to be humiliating to F. This humiliation was also further added to when M changed the subject (from being reprimanded) by referring to F's likeness to her mother in a provocative, almost mocking manner. He then seemed to hold his dominance when he authoritatively refers to himself as 'mixed-race' and to his brother as 'brown'. It does not seem surprising that this leads to F bringing up M's father. On the face of it, it seems M is talking about his identity as a boy of Afro-Caribbean descent and perhaps making statements of facts about other people's skin colour. To us, however, it felt that he was at the same time desperate to defend himself and not seem too 'black' and definitely not as brown as his younger brother. I introduced the question about the skin colours of the therapists in a move of relational reflexivity in order to normalise differences in skin colour and through this to attempt to help M out of the painful pattern in which he and his mother were stuck. This pattern was a kind of schismogenesis in which F was unable to relate to M as a child, which led M to feel anxious, uncontained and aggressive, which in turn led to F being further unable to respond.

In this section, I have tried to show how my colleague and I used ideas about correspondence and joining as a process in order to get alongside M and his mother and how by using systemic psychotherapy enquiry techniques such as circular questions, hypothesising and relational reflexivity we attempted to get inside the in-between of their relationship. We learnt something new about aspects of their relationship, although the pattern of push and pull between them (schismogenesis) was repeated.

The life of 'culture' in systemic psychotherapy

What of culture and race in this work? Clearly any aspect of relationships can be implicated in schismogenesis, but would these aspects be driving forces? M's emotional outlook cannot be separated from him being a 13-year-old boy of Afro-Caribbean background living in London, nor can we ignore the experience of M and F against the background of colonisation of the West Indies, the slave trade and the subsequent recruitment of labour from these territories (Gilroy, 1992; Hall, 2017). However, the multi-layering and intricate connections between emotional, cognitive, cultural and social processes, which this work exemplified, are frequently lost in systemic psychotherapists' approaches to clinical work. Perhaps it is fair to say that while correspondence is emphasised, ethnographic details are ignored. Instead, contemporary systemic psychotherapists could be said to be preoccupied with 'culture' as a kind of abstract difference. Despite 'culture' being firmly embedded in the roots of the models for systemic psychotherapy in the form of ethnographic details, the idea was ignored as the discipline took off as a model of psychotherapy, and an interest in 'culture' did not re-emerge until the more recent acknowledgement of the roles of gender and power and a move to a 'second order' orientation placed the systemic psychotherapist as a participant rather than an observer of the system in the therapy room. While this increased interest in social contexts, it did not ignite an interest in accessing anthropological publications or to a return to Bateson's ethnography. Rather, the work carried out in this period tended to describe behaviour, institutions and sometimes family systems of immigrant communities either in the USA or in Great Britain (for example, McGoldrick, Giordano, & Pearce, 1996) with a somewhat essentialising and stereotyping emphasis on diversity from the position of dominant Euro-American professional traditions.

Recently, in tune with the current zeitgeist, this has developed into a different and extremely influential approach in the UK. This is the approach referred to as The Social Grrraacceeesss (Burnham, 1993, 2012; Rober-Hall, 1998; Burnham & Harris, 2002). Here 'culture' is conceptualised in terms of an individual person's right to an identity and this identity being expressed in a myriad differences and diversities. This approach is taught on all systemic psychotherapy foundational courses and is referred to as a kind of 'competence' in assessments. The idea of The Social Grrraacceeesss began as a mnemonic called 'DISGRRACCE' (Disability, I, Sexuality, Gender, Race, Religion, Age, Class, Culture, Ethnicity); John Burnham, a well-known systemic psychotherapist who developed it with colleagues, describes how the aim was to remind himself of processes of discrimination.

> In a teaching session I might put the mnemonic across the top of the board as a visual context/guideword for myself and the participants.
>
> *(Burnham, 2012, p. 140)*

Given the emphasis in second order systemic psychotherapy on individuals in their relationships, their choices and co-construction in the moments of the therapeutic encounter, and the accompanying systemic psychotherapeutic aversion towards the weight of unconscious dispositions, it is easy to understand why the addressing of difference and diversity has taken place within the frame of identity politics and in line with popular and official preoccupations. In a recent publication, Burnham himself has further developed the approach by looking at the mnemonic from positions of four quadrants constructed by two axes, a horizontal one from voiced to unvoiced and a vertical one from visible to invisible (Burnham, 2012, p. 146). For example, from the visible/unvoiced position, visible aspects in the room such as a religious symbol worn by a person may not be mentioned or talked about. Burnham himself suggests that the most difficult quadrant is the invisible/unvoiced quadrant and that perhaps there are some issues in the 'taken for granted' experience of clients about which therapists best refrain from enquiring about (Burnham, 2012).

This approach is problematic. For example, the very idea of a list begs the question of the relationship between the different items on the list, between the different members of the category, in this case, the 'list of differences'. Unless we think of all the items in the list as being of the same order, this list presents a muddle. Do we want to consider 'culture' of the same order as 'age' and 'gender'? What are 'culture' and 'ethnicity' in this list? How can this list be used in practice? Burnham clearly thinks that there is a relationship between the different items on the list, when he suggests that the mnemonic may also be conceptualised as a 'collidescope', which conveys "non-symmetrical, sometimes colliding visions of relations between socially produced differences" (Burnham, 2012, p. 144). If this refers to intersectionality (hooks, 2014; Butler, 2007), that is to say the way differences intersect at particular points in time for particular individuals and at particular locations, this may be a more constructive starting point, but as a technique The Social Grrraacceeesss do not encourage trainees to interrogate these intersections except in a piecemeal and fragmented way. 'Culture' then, has, as Strathern suggests, been 'trivialised' while at other times, when clinicians are making claims to fulfill outcome expectations with respect to multi-cultural client populations, 'culture' (or 'race') becomes 'aggrandised' (Strathern, 1995). This approach to 'culture', then, generally discourages a consideration of historical and institutional connections and relationships, some of which may be outside the awareness of individual persons but nevertheless constitute the background to and are implicated in experience and the way life is lived. It is as if in either case no particular ethnographic details matter and "culture has become recontextualised" (Strathern, 1995).

Da Cunha has distinguished two notions of culture, namely 'culture', the "units in an inter-ethnic system (the reflexive position which speaks about itself)"; and culture, "the more or less shared meanings in external/internal schemes" (Da Cunha, 2009, p. 70). While most anthropologists may accept the latter notion at least as a shorthand of how we define this term, "the reflexive position which speaks about itself" is a fitting description of this re-contextualisation; it captures very well both the phenomenon and the activity we refer to as psychotherapy and accords with contemporary systemic psychotherapy thinking about the co-construction, narratives and dialogue generally as well as with thinking behind the 'Social Grrraacceeesss'. One goes to therapy in order to speak about oneself, with someone else, and in contemporary systemic psychotherapy of second order approaches, this is aimed at personal choice and the therapist working towards realising this for the client. Referring to Foucault's final five lectures (Foucault, 2008), McFalls and Pandolfi conclude that for Foucault this therapeutic mode of government is a particular feature of our present time. This is

> one that legitimises its authority with claims of benevolence, of expertise, and even of empowerment of those whose conduct it guides. Whether it be civil society or the entrepreneurial individual, the neoliberal subject ideally takes charge of its life through a panoply of practices of the self from self-help and self-reliance to self-marketing and self-governance.
>
> *(McFallow & Pandolfi, 2014, p. 173)*

In these circumstances, we may wonder whether psychotherapists and anthropologists are able to hear what clients speak about when we think they speak about 'culture'. Are they speaking for themselves or for someone else or for something else of which they may be a part but which is not the same as themselves? Are they speaking about their relationships? And if so, what do we take this to mean?

The challenge of relationships

One way of defining systemic psychotherapy is to describe it as an approach, which looks for or examines relationships and relationships between relationships as these occur both in the therapy room as well as in the lives of clients and therapists. This is a complex task. Firstly, because the immediate focus is on the persons and their relationships in the therapy room. Not unlike for an ethnographer in the immediacy of a fieldwork encounter, what you see and what you are participating in become where you start. The therapist is interested in the relationships between these persons as well as the relationships between these relationships as they emerge in the room. This includes being curious also about the relationships of each person to others (not in the room) and their relationships with each other and with others in the past and, eventually, about potential relationships which might emerge in the future. It also includes the relationships between the therapist herself and different family members as well as her relationships with others and the relationships between these relationships. Along with social anthropologists, systemic psychotherapists think about these relationships as 'context', a central idea in the discipline (in the UK, a popular magazine called *Context* is published by the Association for Family Psychotherapists), which originally referred to relationships and the interactions and messages exchanged between them; these constituted the context for other messages and relationships. In practice a therapy session and in particular the initial therapy sessions present a challenge precisely because of the presence of several persons and the number of relationships in which each person is implicated. For example, it will not do, when finishing a session, that only one member feels heard, while the others think that they have wasted their time or, worse, feel angry with the therapist because she was not on their side (this is what systemic psychotherapists mean when they talk about 'neutrality' (Selvini Palazzoli et al., 1980; Cecchin, 1987). The systemic psychotherapist therefore aims to join and engage all family members at the outset, without ever having the full picture or context about the family or about the nature or extent of conflicts or problems the family members might be experiencing. Yet, she works with the assumption that the relationships and the way these are represented and expressed in the room are circumscribed or restrained by other relationships, about which she does not know much, if anything. In terms familiar to anthropologists, Strathern describes a parallel from modernist social anthropology with a comment on 'context':

> while contexts shaped the knowledge which the ethnographer derived from seeing something as 'belonging' to this or that social domain, the

> phenomenon in question were not themselves completely encompassed – they always had other dimensions to them.
>
> *(Strathern, 1995, p. 160)*

Working in this way assumes that there always are differences in relationships and between relationships and negotiating these without ever necessarily arriving or stopping at similarities or differences. The aim is to find a way of being curious so that all participants find out something new. So, for example, in the session described above we learnt that F had brought M along using some (small) threat, and F learnt that M had not known that she had tried to do something to improve the relationship, too. The sequence moved in and out of connections and disconnections, and eventually we could discern a repeat of a previous pattern which I and my colleague understood as pivotal to the unhappiness of M and his family.

The global – the local

Bateson described schismogenesis (symmetrical and complementary) twice. First in the 1939 postscript to the *Naven* volume and then again in 1958 after he had become interested in cybernetics.

In 1939 he considered schismogenesis to be

> a process of differentiation in the norms of individual behaviour resulting from cumulative interaction between individuals.
>
> *(Bateson, 1958, p. 175)*

And, in 1958,

> an implicit recognition that the system contains an extra order of complexity due to the combination of learning with the interactions of persons. The schismogenic unit is a two person subsystem. This subsystem contains the potentialities of a cybernetic circuit which might go into progressive change; it cannot therefore be conceptually ignored and must be described in a language of a higher type than any language used to describe individual behaviour.
>
> *(Bateson, 1958, p. 297)*

I have elsewhere described the difference between the two definitions as one between levels of abstraction (Krause, 2012). In the second definition, Bateson included the process of learning, and any interacting and communicating persons learning to learn as they engage in relationships. It seems to me that Batson was referring to an incommensurability between the levels of individual persons in a relationship, on the one hand, and this relationship as this emerges though the process of its own dynamic, on the other, and that this latter meaning is best captured by the concept of 'relationality'. In the paper by Strathern already referred to, she makes a similar observation about the 'global':

> For what is perceived as intractable must lie 'outside' this relational practice, precisely in order to be precipitated and produced by it. The same intellectual activity that connects disparate things also established their separateness. Thus the comparative method does not just create the divisions it overcomes; it also produces anthropologists' very perception of social relations as given. There is a sense, then, in which relationality lies beyond the relational practice of anthropological enquiry.
>
> *(Strathern, 1995, pp. 166–167)*

Strathern prefers the term 'sociality' as an epithet for the global and consequently encourages social anthropologists to study social relations, including 'culture' as a relation, "for they are visibly less than the awareness with which they are used, less than the sociality that brings them into existence" (Strathern, 1995, p. 170).

In psychotherapy, both because of the history which all branches of psychotherapy share, but also because of the embeddedness of practitioners in a totalising and systematic system of knowledge, relations expressed in the clinic, in the hospital and in the therapy room are most often conceived of in universal terms, as if they are 'direct' or uniform expressions of 'relationality' or 'sociality'. In psychoanalytic psychotherapy, this tends to be expressed in terms of the universality of the Oedipus Complex or of the developmental as well as existential denotation of schizoid and depressive positions (Klein, 1946). The two levels do not tend to be distinguished by systemic psychotherapists, either, but for opposite reasons. Being focused on 'abstract differences', systemic psychotherapists tend to be reluctant to engage with what practitioners in the discipline assume persons may actually have in common, apart from the general acceptance that relationships, and relationships between them, are ubiquitous (Krause, 2009). Thus, while psychoanalytically trained practitioners tend to assume that similarities (for example between therapists and clients) are relatively straightforward to access, systemic psychotherapists tend to be reluctant to engage with the idea of similarities theoretically and not to be transparent about the similarities they assume exist between themselves and their clients. This means that there is a tendency to conflate the 'local' with the 'global' and hence to direct the therapy towards individual choice. Anderson and Goolishan, writers well known for having developed the constructionist approach in the discipline, refer to this:

> The process of questions generated from the position of 'not-knowing' results in the development of a locally (dialogically) constructed understanding and a local (dialogic) vocabulary. Local refers to the language, the meaning, and the understanding developed between persons in dialogue, rather than broadly held cultural sensibilities.
>
> *(Anderson & Goolishan, 1992, p. 33)*

The position of the therapist

So far, I have indicated that systemic psychotherapists work with a processual framework, taking account of observations of what happens in time, and particularly during very small sections of time. Relationships are encompassed by other relationships, and what happens at one point has an influence on what happens subsequently. Ingold exemplified this with what he calls a 'dwelling perspective' referring to what people build, either in imagination or on the ground, arise from within their ongoing and involved collective activity rather than the other way around 'We build and have built because we dwell' (Ingold, 2000, 186). This implies attunement not just to content and meaning but also to the *process* through which each of us access, understand, build and perceive. For the systemic psychotherapist this is referred to as 'reflexivity' and has become *the* concept in the discipline, corresponding to ideas of 'transference and countertransference' in psychoanalysis (Bland, 2009; Cooper, 2009; Donovan, 2009). This includes the idea that one is performing and, at the same time, being audience to one's own performance (Tomm, 1987a, 1987b), as well as the idea of talking about talking or thinking about thinking (Burnham, 2005). Thus, in the extract of the therapy session above, we asked M a reflexive question, namely what does he think about our sessions (talking about talking).

Awareness of reflexivity is not new to social anthropologists, as references to Bateson and Ingold suggest, but Rabinow and Stavrianakis further observe that,

> as presently constituted, to our knowledge, none of the institutionalised modes of knowledge of the contemporary disciplines has come to terms adequately with its own conditions of production as essentially contributory to its knowledge claims . . . we are arguing that knowledge claims that systematically rule out reflection on their own modes of governance and habits are wilfully blind to fundamental conditions that make their practice possible.
>
> *(Rabinow & Stavrianakis, 2013, p. 87)*

Elsewhere, I have argued that systemic psychotherapists need to develop a comprehensive reflexivity. This is a reflexivity which encompasses recursiveness between different aspects of meaning, interpretation, and experience held or expressed by persons (either clients or therapists) *as well as* the reflexivity of both the therapist and clients *vis-à-vis* their own history, development and background and the contexts in which they participate (Krause, 2012). The term 'comprehensive reflexivity' is perhaps somewhat clumsy even if it is descriptive, but I believe it was an attempt to capture what Rabinow and Stavrianakis call 'operational perspectivity', noting that "experience is necessarily perspectival relative to the operational capabilities of an agent; but this is not to say that it is necessarily subjective" (Burke, cited in Rabinow & Stavrianakis, 2016, p. 417). This highlights not only the situatedness of experiences but also the instability and potential conflict in situations. I would argue that this is a description of what my colleague and I began to do in the sequence presented in the extract above when we used what is emerging in the therapy session to refer to ourselves. We included ourselves in the hope of beginning to find a way in which our personal and professional background could be explicitly implicated in the knowledge we were producing in our sessions. The markers of skin colour and race were not only alive in our session but were also alive in the clinic where M was allocated to A, because, we suspect, of a perception that they are both 'black'. By including ourselves, we are acknowledging the salience of 'race' to all of us in this context, and of course it also emerges that I am a white woman like M's grandmother, whereas A, who is the only man present in this session and in fact in all our sessions with this family, is a black man a bit like M's father. We are talking about political and emotional ramifications of relationships, but we are, even if somewhat obliquely, also talking about history and about 'culture'. These relationships are positioned between the intractable or non-discursive 'sociality', on the one hand, and the experience of M, F, myself and A of our relationships in the consulting room, on the other. I take Rabinow's and Marcus's idea of 'the contemporary' to refer to just this:

> Thus, if one no longer assumes that the new is what is dominant, to use Raymond Williams's distinction, and that the old is somehow residual, then the question of how older and newer elements are given form and worked together, either well or poorly, becomes a significant site of inquiry. I call that site the contemporary.
>
> *(Rabinow & Marcus, 2008, p. 3)*

The contemporary is specifically situated and therefore produces situated knowledge. While systemic psychotherapists (for reasons I have described above) on the whole have not been very good at inquiring into 'the contemporary', this is the kind of knowledge which social anthropologists and especially ethnographers are well placed to document and therefore help bring forth.

Concluding remarks

Systemic psychotherapy and social anthropology share a great deal of ground as well as some history, even if the relationship has been and is at times ambivalent. For me, this ambivalence is articulated in how hard it feels to write to the space between. Because of grounding theory in 'relationships' rather than in individual developmental or psychic processes, systemic psychotherapists are well placed to take account of 'the contemporary', that is to say, of recent social and 'cultural' processes and the restraints and the impact of these on clients as well as on themselves. I have argued that perhaps partly because of the collective ignorance of the roots of the model in the ethnographic work of Bateson, the discipline has struggled to do this and therefore separates the local, that is to say the interaction and communication in the therapy room, from the global, with a default position on a general notion of 'difference'. Consequently, 'culture' refers to the identity of individuals and tends to be represented as something reified and stereotypic in the minds of systemic psychotherapists. The exploration then tends to veer away from both institutional and unconscious aspects of difference. However, I have also argued that precisely because of the emphasis on 'relationships', social anthropologists and ethnographers may have something to learn from the stance and techniques of enquiry used by systemic psychotherapists, because these can assist the enquirer in getting inside the in-between of relationships from a position of 'correspondence' and operational perspectivity. Perhaps the term 'culture' has a role to play in this as a general gloss, although I am not sure. We can call all that we do 'culture', or we can refuse to use this term for any of it, but given the current neo-liberal zeitgeist and the outcome monitoring bureaucracy in which most therapists, practising either in public services or privately, work, the pragmatic effects of 'culture' as a framing device are not free-floating. Personally, I will not be able to avoid using the term as a shorthand for some kind of 'difference', but I am, though, happier with the term 'relationship' as long as therapists and anthropologists alike consider where they stand in terms of identifying what they may consider to be pre-discursive or intractable.

Note

1 Throughout I use 'Naven' to indicate the ethnography written by Bateson, whereas *naven* refers to the ritual described in that ethnography.

References

Anderson, H. & Goolishan, H. (1988). Human systems as linguistic systems: Preliminary and evolving ideas about the implications for clinical theory. *Family Process*, 27 (4): 371–393.

Anderson, H. & Goolishan, H. (1992). The client is the expert: A not-knowing approach to therapy. In: S. McNamee & K. Gergen (Eds.), *Therapy as Social Construction*, 25–39. London: Sage.

Bateson, G. (1935). Culture contact and schizmogenesis. *Man*, 35 (article 199): 178–183.

Bateson, G. (1949). Bali: The value system of a steady state. In: M. Fortes (Ed.), *Social Structure: Studies Presented to A. R. Radcliffe-Brown*, 35–53. Oxford: The Clarendon Press.

Bateson, G. (1958). *Naven: The Culture of the Iatmul People of New Guinea as Revealed Through the "Naven" Ceremonial*. London: Wildwood House.

Bateson, G. (1971). The cybernetic of "self": A theory of alcoholism. *Psychiatry*, 34 (1): 1–18.

Bateson, G. (1972a). Style, grace and information in primitive art. In: G. Bateson, *Steps to an Ecology of Mind*, 128–152. London: Jason Aronson Inc.

Bateson, G. (1972b). *Steps to an Ecology of Mind: Collected Essays in Anthropology, Psychiatry, Evolution, and Epistemology*. London: Jason Aronson Inc.

Bateson, G. (1979). *Mind and Nature: A Necessary Unity.* New York: E.P. Dutton.

Bateson, G., Jackson, D., Hayley, J., & Weakland, J. (1956). Toward a theory of schizophrenia. *Behavioural Science*, 1 (4): 51–64.

Bland, J. (2009). Working with unconscious processes: Psychoanalysis and systemic family therapy. In: C. Flaskas & D. Pocock (Eds.), *Systems and Psychoanalysis: Contemporary Integrations in Family Therapy*, 21–38. London: Karnac.

Boyd-Franklin, N. (1989). *Black Families in Therapy: A Multisystems Approach.* New York: Guilford.

Burnham, J. (1993). Systemic supervision: The evolution of reflexivity in the context of the supervisory relationship. *Human Systems*, 4: 349–381.

Burnham, J. (2005). Relational reflexivity: A tool for socially constructing therapeutic relationships. In: C. Flaskas, B. Mason, & A. Perlesz (Eds.), *The Space Between: Experience, Context, and Process in the Therapeutic Relationship*, 1–18. London: Karnac.

Burnham, J. (2012). Developments in social GRRRAAACCEEESSS: Visible-invisible and voiced-unvoiced. In: I.-B. Krause (Ed.), *Culture and Reflexivity in Systemic Psychotherapy: Mutual Perspectives*, 139–162. London: Karnac.

Burnham, J. & Harris, Q. (2002). Cultural perspectives in supervision. In: D. Campbell & B. Mason (Eds.), *Perspectives on Supervision*, 21–41. London: Karnac.

Butler, J. (2007). *Gender Trouble: Feminism and the Subversion of Identity.* New York & London: Routledge.

Ceechin, G. (1987). Hypothesizing, circularity and neutrality revisited: An invitation to curiosity. *Family Process*, 26: 405–413.

Cooper, A. (2009). Hearing the grass grow: Emotional and epistemological challenges of practice-near research. *Journal of Social Work Practice*, 23 (4): 429–442.

Da Cunha, M. C. (2009). *"Culture" and Culture: Traditional Knowledge and Intellectual Rights.* Chicago: Prickly Paradigm Press.

Dewey, J. (1966). *Democracy and Education: An Introduction to the Philosophy of Education.* New York: Free Press.

Donovan, M. (2009). Reflecting process and reflecting functioning: Shared concerns and challenges in systemic and psychoanalytic therapeutic practice. In: C. Flaskas & D. Pocock (Eds.), *Systems and Psychoanalysis: Contemporary Integrations in Family Therapy*, 149–168. London: Karnac.

Falicov, C. (1995). Training to think culturally: A multidimensional comparative framework. *Family Process*, 34: 389–399.

Foucault, M. (2008). *The Birth of Biopolitics: Lectures at the Collegè de France 1973–1974.* New York: Picador.

Gilroy, R. (1992) [1987]. *There Ain't No Black in the Union Jack.* London & New York: Routledge.

Hall, S. (2017). *Familiar Stranger: A Life Between Two Islands.* London: Allan Lane. (With B. Schwartz).

Harries-Jones, P. (1995). *A Recursive Vision: Ecological Understanding and Gregory Bateson.* Toronto & London: University of Toronto Press.

hooks, b. (2014). *Writing Beyond Race: Living Theory and Practice.* New York & London: Routledge.

Ingold, T. (1986). *Evolution and Social Life.* Cambridge: Cambridge University Press.

Ingold, T. (2000). *The Perception of the Environment: Essays in Livelihood, Dwelling and Skill.* London & New York: Routledge.

Ingold, T. (2017). On human correspondence. *Journal of the Royal Anthropological Institute*, 23 (1): 9–27.

Klein, M. (1946). Notes on some schizoid mechanisms. *International Journal of Psychoanalysis*, 27: 99–110.

Krause, I.-B. (2002). *Culture and System in Family Therapy*. London: Karnac.

Krause, I.-B. (2007). Reading Naven: Toward the integration of culture in systemic psychotherapy. *Human Systems: The Journal of Systemic Consultation and Management*, 18: 112–125.

Krause, I.-B. (2009). In the thick of culture: Systemic and psychoanalytic ideas. In: C. Flaskas & D. Pocock (Eds.), *Systems and Psychoanalysis: Contemporary Integrations in Family Therapy*, 167–184. London: Karnac.

Krause, I.-B. (Ed.) (2012). *Culture and Reflexivity in Systemic Psychotherapy: Mutual Perspectives*. London: Karnac.

Marcus, G. M. (1985). A timely reading of Naven: Gregory Bateson as an oracular essayist. *Representations*, 12: 66–82.

McFalls, L. & Pandolfi, M. (2014). Parrhesia and Therapeusis: Foucault on and in the world of contemporary neoliberalism. In: J. Faubion (Ed.), *Foucault Now: Current Perspectives on Foucault Studies*, 168–187. Cambridge: Polity Press.

McGoldrick, M., Giordano, J., & Pearce, J. K. (Eds.) (1996). *Ethnicity and Family Therapy*. New York: Guilford Press.

Minuchin, S., Montalvo, B., Guerney, B. G., Rosman, B. L., & Schumer, F. (1967). *Families of the Slum: An Exploration of Their Structure and Treatment*. New York: Basic Books.

Nuckolls, C. W. (1996). *The Dialectics of Knowledge and Desire*. Madison, WI: University of Wisconsin Press.

Rabinow, P. & Marcus, G. E. (2008). *Designs for an Anthropology of the Contemporary*. Durham & London: Duke University Press.

Rabinow, P. & Stavrianakis, A. (2013). *Demands of the Day: On the Logic of Anthropological Enquiry*. Chicago, IL: Chicago University Press.

Rabinow, P. & Stavrianakis, A. (2016). Movement space: Putting anthropological theory, concepts and cases to the test. *Hau: Journal of Ethnographic Theory*, 6: 403–431.

Rober-Hall, A. (1998). Working systemically with older people and their families, who have "come to grief". In: P. Sutcliffe, G. Tufnell, & U Cornish (Eds.), *Working with Dying and Bereaved: Systemic Approaches to Therapeutic Work*, 177–206. London: MacMillan.

Selvini Palazzoli, M., Boscolo, L., Cecchin, G., & Prata, G. (1980). Hypothesizing-circularity- neutrality: Three questions for the conductor of the session. *Family Process*, 19 (1): 3–12.

Shotter, J. (2010). *Social Construction on the Edge: "Withness": Thinking & Embodiment*. Chagrin Falls, OH: Taos Institute Publications.

Silverman, E. K. (2001). *Masculinity, Motherhood and Mockery: Psychoanalyzing Culture and the Iatmul Naven Rite of New Guinea*. Ann Arbor, MI: The University of Michigan Press.

Strathern, M. (1995). The nice thing about culture is that everyone has it. In: M. Strathern (Ed.), *Shifting Contexts: Transformations in Anthropological Knowledge*, 153–176. New York & London: Routledge.

Tomm, K. (1987a). Interventive interviewing: Part I. Strategizing as a fourth guideline for the therapist. *Family Process*, 26: 3–13.

Tomm, K. (1987b). Interventive interviewing: Part II. Reflexive questioning as a means to enable self-healing. *Family Process*, 26: 167–183.

4

THERAPY AND THE RISE OF THE MULTICULTURAL

Keir Martin

The rapid growth of a concern regarding 'cultural' sensitivity and difference has been one of the most marked developments in psychotherapy in recent decades. The statistical evidence of the move of an interest in cultural issues from the margin to the centre of academic research in therapy is clear. For example, an initial consultation of the Psychinfo database of published research that I conducted in June 2014 that combines 'counsel(l)ing' or 'therapy' (or some variant thereof, such as 'therapeutic' or 'counsel(l)or') with 'culture' (or a related term, such as 'cultural') in the title provided 946 results and papers in the title. Only one instance of this combination occurs in the first half of the twentieth century. By contrast, five instances of this combination occurred in the first three months of 2014 alone and 160 examples of this combination (17% of the total) appeared in just the three years 2011–2014, and 248 (26%) appeared in the preceding five years. Although part of this clustering might be explained by the current efflorescence of academic publications, it is hard to imagine that this accounts for all of the increase.

Other arenas show a similar growing interest. *Therapy Today* is the house magazine of the British Association for Counselling and Psychotherapy, which in keeping with the BACP's status as the largest psychotherapy accrediting body in the UK is also the nation's most widely distributed professional psychotherapy journal. In recent years, articles discussing cultural competence have become regular features. To take one recent example, April 2016's editorial informs us that a recent, 'large national study of adverse effects of counseling and psychotherapy . . . raises some important points' (Jackson 2016:3). Among over issues, the editorial is largely given over to the finding that certain groups, including 'black and minority ethnic people', are 'more likely to report adverse effects of therapy'. The implications that the reader is expected to draw are clear.

> The finding about BME clients is sobering and, as the researchers say, points to a need for the profession to include much more content on

> cultural awareness in both initial training curricula and continuing professional development. Half a day on 'diversity issues' isn't going to do it.
>
> *(Jackson 2016:3)*

In fact, the implications are not as clear in this case as is claimed. The cited report cautions that the self-reporting of negative impacts can only be taken as evidence for just that – the perception of a negative impact – and that although other research suggests that 5–10% of clients have worse symptoms after treatment, this cannot necessarily be attributed to the treatment itself. The authors themselves point to several limitations in the survey, including 'a low response rate and a reliance on patient recall of information about the type and duration of treatment that they received'. There was also a lack of information about other 'diagnoses or other clinical details'. (Crawford et al. 2016: 263). As a consequence, the report's summary is understated and qualified in terms of its recommendations:

> Our findings may indicate a need to place greater emphasis on the development of therapists' cultural competence during initial training and subsequent professional development activities.
>
> *(Crawford et al. 2016:264)*

This is quite some distance from the definitive claim that 'the researchers say[their research] points to a need for the profession to include much more content on cultural awareness in both initial training curricula' (Jackson ibid.), which is made in the appropriation of their report in *Therapy Today*.

The research has other potential blindsides. Half of its findings relate to the potential for negative outcomes of different kinds of therapy, with the other devoted to an analysis of the extent to which negative outcomes are likely to be reported by particular groups. But there is no comparison for these two sets of data. So, we know the relative possibility of CBT being reported negatively as opposed to humanistic therapy, and the relative possibility of BME clients reporting negatively for therapy in general as opposed to non-BME, but we have no sense of whether the higher reporting rate for particular client groups is consistent across modalities. The majority of respondents (51.03%) reported having received CBT only, raising the possibility that the negative outcomes reported by certain groups are partially connected to this particular modality, but the data gives us no way of knowing. As the main corresponding author informed me in response to a query, although the overall sample was large,

> amounts of data in some cells representing these combinations of therapies and demographics were too small to allow meaningful comparison.
>
> *(Crawford 2017)*

The findings of this research are therefore potentially ambiguous in a number of regards. How that ambiguity is transformed into a definitive moral statement and course of action in the *Therapy Today* editorial is revealing. It suggests that a decision has already been made and a direction of travel has already been decided upon; namely, 'to include much more content on cultural awareness' on training curricula. 'How can a profession claim professional status if it is in denial about its own failures and mistakes?' (Jackson ibid.) concludes the editorial, in a tone that implies that any questioning of this interpretation is a denial not only of reality but moral responsibility, even if, on fairly light closer inspection, in this instance the evidence marshalled in support of this claim is nowhere near as unambiguous as it is presented.

Culture and psychotherapeutic theory

This perspective's underlying framing is one in which traditional psychotherapy is presented as having been blind to the importance of cultural difference, instead imposing an unquestioned universalistic vision based on Western individualism upon humanity. In many regards, this is a long-standing and familiar criticism (see Introduction this volume). Some of the earliest critiques of Freud were based upon a claim that his theories were expressions of the particular culture of his middle-class Viennese milieu that had been inappropriately universalised and that many of the concepts that he claimed were universal aspects of human psychological development, such as the Oedipus complex, were not found or manifested themselves very differently in different cultural contexts (e.g. Malinowski 1927). In the decades since, other theorists seem to have been more than willing to encourage this impression, with even more open dismissals of the potential importance of cultural difference. So, for example Berne (1975:323), the founder of Transactional Analysis, argued that

> culture has very little to do with scripts. There are winners and losers in every layer of society and in every country, and they go about fulfilling their destinies in much the same way all over the world.

And it remains the case that many schools of therapy (particularly more traditional psychoanalytic or psychodynamic schools of therapy) remain resistant to claims that they should integrate cultural difference into their analysis or training. It also remains the case that many still tend to see references to the importance of cultural factors as sophisticated forms of intellectual defence mechanisms designed to resist the real work of therapy, as for example the claim by Elise Snyder, the Chair of the 'China America Psychoanalytic Alliance', that when 'patients' reference their 'culture', it is a classic avoidance technique. 'Clearly, this is a resistance . . . patients would rather talk about their cultures than themselves' (Snyder 2014:94).

However, while 'culture' has definitely become a more central part of therapeutic discourse in recent decades, the idea that earlier generations of therapists were entirely unconcerned with cultural context or cultural difference is slightly misleading. For example, Erikson (1977[1951]) devotes two chapters of his book *Childhood and Society* to an analysis of the importance of understanding cultural differences among two North American native groups, and the rest of the book is replete with references to the importance of understanding cultural difference. Even Freud, who has often been cast as a simple universalist, was on occasion profoundly aware of and concerned to explore the meaning and importance of cultural difference. It is true that culture frequently appears in Freud's writings as an achievement resulting from the renunciation or conquest of natural instinctual drives, but it does not necessarily follow from this that he viewed this process and its outcomes as preordained by the natural constitution of human instinct. His discussions of the relationship between modernity and neurosis bear testament to that. In the *Three Essays on the Theory of Sexuality*, for example, we find the claim that an important, if often overlooked, factor in the development of neurosis is

> the preponderance attaching to in mental life to memory-traces in comparison with recent impressions. This factor is clearly dependent on intellectual education and increases in proportion to the degree of individual culture. The savage has been described in contrast as 'das ungluckselige Kind des Augenblickes' (the hapless child of the moment). In consequence of the inverse relation holding between civilization and the free development of sexuality, of which the consequences can be followed far into the structure of our existences, the course taken by the sexual life of a child is just as unimportant for later life where the cultural or social level is relatively low as it is important where that level is relatively high.
>
> *(Freud 1991[1905]:168)*

Freud's depiction of childlike savages existing at a lower cultural level to civilised man is unlikely to find many adherents in today's cultural climate. But it does nuance what is almost universally considered to be a central tenet of Freud's universal theory of human development and nature: the importance of childhood development and repressed memories of sexuality as an instinctual force in this period. Here we are told that in fact this is a culturally determined phenomenon just as much as it is the intra-psychic factor that leads to the development of the higher cultural achievements of civilised man. In this passage, at least, Freud seems to display a keen awareness of how cultural difference might shape the very core of human nature.

The literature teems with other examples where contemporary critics seem unaware that that those that they are criticising were fully aware of the cultural aspects of the phenomena that they were exploring. For example, Rogers is often held to account for universalising a particular validation of individual freedom and self-development that was blind to its cultural roots and its potential inapplicability or lack of appeal to those from other cultural contexts. We see this very clearly in the influential work of John McLeod, for example (see Introduction this volume). But it's clear that Rogers was keenly aware of the roots of his own theoretical revolution in the particular historical moment of the development of American culture within which he was writing. To take one of a number of acknowledgments of this from his own work:

> It is a product of its time and cultural setting. . . . Some of its roots stretch out even further into the educational and social and political philosophy which is at the heart of our American culture. . . . Thus client-centered therapy has drawn, both consciously and unconsciously, upon many of the current streams of cultural, scientific, and philosophical thought which are present in our culture.
>
> *(Rogers 1951:4–5)*

Interestingly here, Rogers demonstrates the same distinction between 'culture' and 'culture' that is a problematic feature of much 'cultural' analysis in contemporary psychotherapy. Culture is ultimately everywhere if one accepts it as a useful concept, and ultimately nothing lies outside of it. But in order for it to be *used* as a concept in most contexts, some features of culture have to be separated out from the rest of 'culture' and then defined as the particular 'culture' under discussion. Rather than accepting any such particular separation as definitive, the far more important work, ethnographically and therapeutically, is the attempt to understand what work it is doing in separating out some aspects of 'culture' from the rest of the 'culture' in order to create an object defined as 'culture' that can be worked with in particular ways in particular contexts. The ethnographer of contemporary psychotherapy might do this with the ways in which 'culture' is discussed in training manuals without necessarily wishing to dismiss or accept any particular framing, instead attempting, for example, to understand the work that this linguistic separation performs in order to shape a new 'professional' body of psychotherapists. The therapist might wish to do this with a client's shifting references to their 'culture' without accepting either that there is a culture exactly as it is referred to in any instance outside of that evocation or, conversely, that such evocation is simply bad faith or a resistance to the 'real' issues. Again, what is therapeutically interesting is the work that is done by that linguistic evocation in that particular moment.

Hence, Rogers (op cit:5) goes on to say that not everything is 'culture' and that it would be 'a mistake to view client-centered therapy as solely a product of cultural influences'. By this, he means those elements of US mid-twentieth-century 'culture' that underpinned his vision. Like McLeod, Rogers was aware of the particular historical cultural context of elements of his own thought. In a meeting that I had with McLeod in Oslo in 2017, he expressed some surprise that Rogers had written this when I mentioned it to him. This is an interesting lacuna, given McLeod's justified reputation as a leading theorist and scholar of psychotherapy and person-centred therapy in particular. One of the sessions on person-centred therapy in my training course, for example, was dedicated to McLeod's work along with that of Mick Cooper, under the heading of the 'New Pluralism'. Yet the lacuna is perhaps revealing, as any therapist or ethnographer would expect. The current promotion of 'culture' perhaps requires that our therapeutic predecessors be constructed as 'culture-blind' in order for the contemporary addition of a particular model of 'culture' to take root.

Rogers himself appears to be looking for something universal in human behaviour illuminated by his approach that goes beyond the 'culture' of the 1950s USA. But this universal element in human being is not simply the expression of the 'bounded individualism' that McLeod argues unites all 'psychological' therapies from Freud onwards. Instead, Rogers (ibid.) is explicit that his theory is

> built upon close, intimate, and specific observations of man's behavior in a relationship . . . which it is believed transcend to some degree the limitations or influences of a given culture.

For Rogers, it is human behaviour in relationships that is fundamental to human being, and it is this fundamental aspect of being that transcends *particular historic cultures*. Hence the word 'culture' here for Rogers does the work of separating out those aspects of particular relational webs, within which persons come into being, from the general universal importance of relationality (to use contemporary terminology), not a general sense of the outside and relational to be opposed to the interior of the bounded individual, as with McLeod's constructions.

Talking about the emergence of the kind of fluid model of individual personhood that he saw emerging from the kind of therapy that he was advocating, he asks:

> Would everyone agree that this is a desirable model of change, that it moves in valued directions? I believe not. . . . This will be one of the social value judgments which individuals and cultures will have to make.
>
> *(Rogers 1961:155)*

Indeed, the more one looks through the historic literature, the more one finds that references to the importance of cultural factors far outweigh dismissals such as Berne's. I take one more example at random, simply as the last therapy-related book that I read for non-academic purposes. Alice Miller, coming from a more classical psychoanalytic tradition than Rogers, is also keen to stress that the person treated by contemporary psychotherapy is not a universal expression of human nature, but herself a particular cultural phenomenon.

> Depression is a disease of our time. Within a culture that was shielded from other value systems, such as that of orthodox Jewry in the ghetto, or of Negro families in the Southern states a hundred years ago, an adapted individual was not autonomous and did not have his own individual sense

> of identity (in our sense) that could have given him support; but he did feel supported by the group. . . . Today it is hardly possible for any group to remain so isolated from others who have different values. Therefore it is necessary today for the individual to find support within himself.
>
> *(Miller 1990[1979]:59)*

Again, there is much in the language used here and in the depiction of bounded cultural groups (even if they are here acknowledged as a historical phenomenon) that cuts against contemporary anthropological understandings of culture. But underlying it is a keen awareness that the kind of individualism that psychotherapy is often criticised for universalising is itself a highly specific cultural product. And, as we shall see, this vision of anti-individualist bounded collective cultures that many anthropologists would find problematically stereotyping with reference to 'Negro families in the Southern States' or 'orthodox Jewry in the ghetto' is remarkably close to the vision of 'Asian' and other non-Western 'cultures' towards which contemporary therapy trainees are expected to perform adherence as a sign of their cultural sensitivity and respect for diversity.

The incorporation of culture

The addition of an awareness of 'culture' is not as novel a trend in psychotherapy as some of its current adherents seem to imagine. What is novel, perhaps, is the work that this concept is being asked to do. It is now increasingly used as a conceptual tool that helps to shape 'best practice' within an increasingly 'professionalized' discipline. It is the desire to use 'culture' as a tool to this end that in large part determines the particular conceptualisation of 'culture' that therapy has adopted. It is a model of culture that is itself just as much a product of a specific historical cultural moment as the kind of 'individualism' held up to scrutiny by Miller. As one unusually nuanced recent article in *Therapy Today* observes, the model of 'culture' being used is one that has become 'a contentious concept in anthropology', being based largely on the kind of totalising, shared and self-replicating model that the discipline has largely discarded in the past three decades (Cameron 2017:32).

That that model is alive and well in contemporary therapeutic applications of 'culture', despite its rejection within anthropology, is easy to demonstrate. In my own training as a therapist, this was the working understanding of 'culture' that dominated discussion of the issue. The handout for the first session on the topic on our course illustrated the framing perfectly. The heading 'Issues of Race and Culture in Counselling' (Jenkins 2011) itself is suggestive of the implicit association of 'culture' with racial or ethnic Otherness that underpins these discussions. This is followed by a list of 'Definitions'.

Culture: 'the shared history, practices, beliefs and values of a racial, regional or religious group of people' (d'Ardenne and Mahtani 1999:4).

Transcultural counselling: 'Counsellors in this setting are responsible for working across, through or beyond their cultural differences' (d'Ardenne and Mahtani 1999:5).

Multicultural counselling: 'an integrative approach that draws upon ideas and techniques from existing theories of counselling, and builds them into a culture-informed and culture-sensitive model of practice' (McLeod 2003:268).

These definitions clearly articulate the model of 'culture' as the 'shared' objective property and essence of a bounded 'group' of people that has already been discussed. The basis of this model is an attempt to overcome the assumed culture-blind individualism of Western culture (and by extension of Western therapy), which is then clearly articulated in the following list of 'Potential cultural barriers to understanding'.

- Ethnocentric models of counselling and change.
- Focus on individual autonomy, rather than on community responsibility.
- Role expectations of counsellor (as expert and adviser, rather than facilitator?).

The underlying framing is clearly articulated here: counselling and therapy tend to focus on an ethnocentric model that focuses on individual autonomy, and this will be a barrier to cross-cultural understanding with clients from other backgrounds, who will give greater priority to 'community responsibility'. It is worth noting here that the focus on 'community responsibility' is a particular framing of the 'culture' argument. It is possible to put forward an argument for taking an individual person's cultural context seriously that does not mean prioritising 'community responsibility' over 'individual autonomy', as if they were automatically a zero-sum game. Indeed, it could be argued that this particular framing of 'community' versus 'individual' is itself a particularly 'Western' cultural perspective, as was argued by anthropological theorists from Ruth Benedict onwards. A framing that conflates cultural awareness with responsibility to the 'community' is probably not a surprising outcome of the model of culture taken from thinkers like Benedict, however, which views 'culture' as a shared history or pattern of beliefs. It does leave unanswered, however, the question of who defines the boundaries of the 'community' – who gets to define who has which legitimate responsibilities to it and what we do with those whose emotional needs are considered incompatible with the official depiction of the 'culture' formalised by its most powerful members.

Other course material framed cultural issues in a similar manner. One article from *Therapy Today* that was written by a UK therapist of South Asian ethnic origin and circulated as a handout informed the reader that

> the British South Asian culture is very traditional: if the individual is experiencing any difficulty, then they are expected to consult the eldest

> member of the family first and if this doesn't help then the religious leaders. They will not access any Western help unless a problem becomes really severe because of *izzat* – the shame it would bring on the entire family – and the fear of becoming the subject of gossip in the community.
>
> *(Khan 2013:21)*

This stark opposition between 'traditional culture' and 'Western help' clearly serves a useful purpose for the author in this context in helping him to express a general difference in attitude and being that he has reason to believe will be largely unfamiliar to the largely white audience he imagines as the readership of his article. In this regard, it fulfils a similar useful purpose to variants of the 'in my culture' trope, which clients from a variety of backgrounds have used in the therapy room in an attempt to describe to me aspects of daily life that they imagine would seem unproblematic to those who in that context might be seen as being of a 'shared' background, but that need to be explicitly illuminated for me. But the danger is that such stark statements are taken as further evidence for a framing that somehow suggests 'South Asians' are as incapable of 'individualism' as 'Westerners' are allegedly incapable of 'community responsibility'. Do all members of the 'culture' feel equally attached to all such traditions at all times? Or do they potentially feel ambiguously attached to and rejecting of them – much as the client described in Rogers' (1961:100) account is ambiguously expressing a desire for autonomy that fits the zeitgeist of 1950s USA while rejecting its consumerism, which she sees as being a force for conformity as much as for individual self-expression. We are all capable of ambiguity towards the (cultural) contexts in which we find ourselves. Khan's own piece deftly illustrates the conflicts within 'cultures' and persons in relation to 'their culture' with his subsequent discussion of the particular pressures that he had to follow particular kinds of careers as someone from an 'upper-class' family. A fluid model of cultural competence might explore the ambiguous feelings, positive and negative, that clients feel towards the environments they find themselves in and the ways in which they evoke an entity called 'culture' in order to make sense of and communicate that ambiguity to others. Once those particular evocations become frozen and reified into fixed objects that assume, for example, that West = individual and non-West = community, then they have the capacity to do as much harm as models that assume that the universal model of humanity is one in which everyone should want to become a particular kind of 'bounded individual'. Such a framing potentially leaves us deaf to those instances when clients begin to tentatively explore their frustrations with 'community responsibility' or the demands of 'shame' in the room with us, as we go into the encounter imagining that our textbooks and power-point slides have already armed us with the knowledge of what 'individuality' means to them, that 'individuality' is not what they want or, worse, that it is ultimately not good for them.

This underlying model of cultural difference continued to underpin discussions throughout other sections of the course outside of the sections explicitly earmarked for culture and diversity issues. For example, there was a strong emphasis on learning how to read, evaluate and conduct academic research on the course. This was part of the general trend towards 'evidence-based' practice that we were told was required by funders and employers, in which insight allegedly gained by personal experience in a therapeutic situation or individual reflection was unlikely to be considered seriously as evidence. Hence, a large amount of time on the course was devoted to these concerns, with less time devoted to practices designed to develop personal sensibilities in therapy practice, such as case-discussion sessions, than in other courses that older colleagues of mine had taken in previous decades. This too was part of a wider trend in which the learning of particular skills and competencies that could be measured and audited took increasing space. So, for example, in the second year, there were twenty-one sessions on professional practice, including issues such as career development and legal safeguards. There were six sessions on research, covering such issues as 'evidence-based practice'. Socio-cultural context was also now considered to be a core component, taking up eleven sessions, with one or two sessions devoted to each of the check-list of factors designed to demonstrate that the course had covered all the bases; gender – check; race – check; disability – check; sexual orientation – check; religion – check and so on. It is worth noting that this way of operating fits a more general trend in which issues are increasingly separated out from the person to be analysed and treated as partially separate objects of analysis. This is of a piece with the increasing trend in training to look at specific 'treatments' for specific kinds of 'client issues'. Despite the good intentions, it can add to the sense that these are boxes to tick through an appreciation of a set of abstractions presented in power point or textbooks rather than understood anew in their meaning in each encounter with another. And it is worth noting also that the place of socio-cultural factors alongside other such learning of particular factors comes at the direct expense of the cultivation of such abilities on the curriculum. The direct discussion of case work was described to me by older colleagues as a process in which their skill and ability to make sense of how such factors played out inside themselves and in relation with clients incrementally increased over the course of their training due to its weekly nature, and hence was at the core of their development as practitioners. In the second year of our course, when most of us were in the heart of our first experience of real practice with clients, there were a grand total of five sessions devoted to the actual discussion of this case material. Given that there were eight people to a group, it was entirely possible for a person to qualify without more than a few minutes' discussion of one of their actual client cases.

The material that we discussed in the section of the course designed to teach us the importance of evaluating 'evidence-based' research illustrated the prevailing conception of 'culture' perfectly. In one exercise, we were separated into four groups and given different published research articles to evaluate. Mine was on issues of culture and diversity, and the main text illustrated the by now hegemonic conception of 'culture' that trainees were broadly expected to perform acknowledgment of. The paper focuses on 'acculturation and ethnic identity in marginal immigrant South Asian men in Britain' and raises a number of important issues as to the specific experiences of this group and their relationship to therapeutic services. 'Culture' and 'acculturation' are the key framings used to understand this experience. 'Acculturation' refers to the process of being 'unable to affiliate and relate to their own ethnic or host culture' (Dhillon and Ubhi 2006:43). From the start, it should be noted that the model of 'culture' used here is one of separable discrete and unified systems (*the* 'host' culture and '*their own* ethnic culture') that are also in some way separate from the person themselves, who then has to attempt to successfully relate to them. Being trapped between the two leaves a person potentially tragically unable to relate to either. This is described in a manner strikingly reminiscent of anthropologist Ruth Benedict's (1934:22) famous depiction of her Native American 'Digger' informant, trapped 'between two cultures whose values and ways of thought were incommensurable'. This is a depiction that anthropologists today largely eschew precisely on the basis that it presents cultures as discrete objects external to the persons who are moulded by them, rather than seeing culture as a fluid process constantly remade and recreated in the ongoing interaction between persons. There is no doubt that clients often experience the world in this way, that the language they can use to make sense of their experience is that of being caught between cultures. Dhillon and Ubhi (2006) give some beautiful examples of this in their paper, and it is my own experience of working with a variety of clients (including some from apparently conventionally 'Western' backgrounds). This is 'culture' as a heuristic trope for the client to make sense of experience that is hence being discursively recreated in each utterance. Each evocation of 'culture' will refer to something slightly different from the last, and this is precisely what a therapist should be most attentive to. This is different, however, from a conception of 'culture' as something objectively 'out there' as an object to which we relate. Again, we can all experience 'culture' in this manner, and sometimes it is useful to make sense of our experience in these terms, but the slippage between these two senses and the consequent objectification of culture is characteristic of how the term is used in this and most similar texts. In this text, culture is repeatedly discussed in this 'objective' manner, often with reference to earlier anthropological texts. Hence, at one point the reader is informed that

> the role of culture in determining an individual's identity is therefore crucial, as the individual's sense of identity is derived from the culture they exist within.
>
> *(Douglas and Isherwood 1979)*

The distinction between immigrant culture and Western culture is drawn in the stark terms that we have already come to expect.

> South Asian culture is typified by a group orientation, where individual needs are subordinated for the good of the group. In contrast, British culture favours the rights of the individual over the group.
>
> *(Dhillon and Ubhi op cit:44)*

It is of course important to be aware of the relational entanglements that both make people what they are and can also be experienced as stopping them from becoming what they might become. It is certainly potentially insensitive to order a client to think of themselves before others and to not take into account the very real relational and emotional barriers to doing that, as one client quoted in this piece describes his therapist as having done. Regardless of the client's 'cultural' background, they will be likely to have such relational entanglements, and there are many therapists who would want to allow the client to explore such issues on their own terms rather than directing to them to reject or submit to such relational pressures. But the very material presented in this paper suggests that on occasion the same South Asian clients who are presented as outcomes of a conformist community-oriented 'culture' are as capable as any 'Western' therapist of rejecting its premises and seeking something that looks very 'individualistic' by contrast. The client who expresses frustration with the therapist, who instructs him to think of himself first, also says,

> I want to, but what I want doesn't matter! (shouting) That would kill me. I have to look after my parents and my younger brother. There are duties.
>
> *(ibid.)*

Another client is quoted as saying that,

> I think our families are too close and interfering. They don't know anything about me. . . . They are always unhappy with me and we fight all the time. I love them but I am trapped in all this. I leave home and come back. I am unhappy and they are unhappy.
>
> *(op cit:45)*

The conclusion that the authors draw from this is that Western therapists should question their 'cultural' assumptions about the nature of the self. We should always be questioning our assumptions, but what strikes me most here is that if there is one thing that the clients here are questioning more than their therapists' blindness to their 'culture', it is their own relationship to that culture and the extent to which it allows them to be the people that they want to be. If there is one 'cultural assumption' of self that these extracts call into question, it is that of Western = individual and non-Western = collective. Here it is the clients who clearly articulate a desire for more individual freedom and autonomy. It is of course entirely possible that the therapist misunderstands the nature of the relational entanglements that make it appear difficult or impossible for the client to move in that direction, and that she could benefit from educating herself more on those barriers (although whether that education is best gained from cultural textbooks or from the client herself is another discussion). But it is clearly not the case that the 'culture' produces selves that either desire absolute autonomy or have no interest in it. Instead, what these extracts demonstrate is something that Rogers might have viewed as something universal: a desire for autonomy *within relationships, not opposed to them.* The nature of the particular relationships with which each client is entangled and the particular challenges that they pose to that desire will vary, and some of those variations may be usefully grouped together under the rubric of 'culture' on occasion. A hypothetical non-Western therapist might be stunned by the extent to which a British client surrenders her autonomy to the demands of paid employment, for example. It is certainly not the case that these extracts simply illustrate the contrast between the Western individual and non-Western collectivist selves that they are intended to illustrate, and that is the basic contrast increasingly drawn in 'cultural' competence training in contemporary psychotherapy.

This framing of 'culture', which I experienced as a trainee, fits a wider zeitgeist of managerial reform of therapy at a national level. My training course was accredited by the BACP, an organisation whose leadership has been promoting a very deliberate policy of 'professionalisation' in recent years. This process has been controversial among many members, some of whom fear that the BACP leadership wishes to transform itself into what would essentially become an outsourced tick-box competence-checking verification service for increasingly centralised and bureaucratically organised state- or employer-provided massified mental health care. The recent rise of 'culture' 'diversity' and 'difference' issues does not just coincide with this agenda; it has been a central part of it. These issues have gone from not being explicitly mentioned in previous versions of the BACP's Ethical Frameworks for Practitioners to being increasingly central components of them. They have become one of the core new professional competencies that practitioners need to perform acknowledgment of, regardless of the multiplicity of perspectives that are actually found in the profession on the subject.

So, for example, the application to become a BACP 'Accredited' practitioner involves writing a section on 'Knowledge and Understanding' on reflexive practice that will be assessed by an examiner. This section has a check-list of three issues that must be mentioned in order to pass this stage.

8.1 Describe a rationale for all your client work with reference to the theory / theories that informs all your practice

(If the theory/theories used did not form part of your practitioner training / CPD evidence, please explain how you came to practise in this way.)

8.2 Describe the place of your self-awareness within your way of working

(This section should describe how you use your reflective awareness of yourself in relation to your understanding of the therapy process.)

8.3 Describe how issues of difference and equality impact upon the therapeutic relationship

(This awareness should also include how you consider issues of difference and equality in the context of your work.) (BACP 2018a:22).

'Difference and equality' in this context is the check-box into which 'culture' is fitted, alongside other issues such as gender or disability. The underlying framing is that the problem this is meant to fix is the therapist's presumed blindness to a particular kind of 'difference' between bounded cultural 'groups'. This is made clear following point from the 2014 guidelines designed to help candidates jump through the hoop successfully.

9.3 How your practice demonstrates your awareness of issues of difference and equality and the impact they have upon your counselling/psychotherapy relationships

Remember, the whole of criterion 9 should be case material, and so you need to explain how your awareness of issues of difference and equality impacted upon the work you did with the client or clients you have chosen to write about. How did your awareness of issues of difference and equality between you and your client affect the way you worked? How did your client/clients perceive themselves in relation to others? What about similarities? How did you guard against being seduced into over identification by apparent similarities between yourself and/or other client groups and so on? (Lloyd 2014:2).

It is revealing that the one danger that is flagged up is the danger of 'being seduced' by 'apparent' similarities. The assumption is that the trap that therapist will fall into is seeing similarities that are not there, to which the antidote is presumably more cultural awareness textbooks and power-points. The logical corollary danger, that the therapist might be seduced into seeing irreconcilable difference by an assumption of 'cultural' difference and blind herself to moments when a client is looking to explore moments of connection with the therapist that begin to break out of normative cultural scripts, is not even mentioned. The desired response is for the trainee to perform one's 'awareness' of the former danger and to ignore the latter.

Other material produced by the BACP continues in a similar vein. BACP provides a number of 'research overview' documents for its members that are available online. The document on 'Equality, diversity and inclusion in the counseling professions' has a section on 'culture' that is largely framed in a similar manner. Hence, at one point members are informed that research shows that 'gender roles are more rigid in Arabic communities' and

> individualism and self-achievement, independence and psychological emancipation from parents and personal identity may not be as important and may be second only to a collectivist outlook, whereby the good of the family, the clan or tribe is put before the good of the individual.
>
> *(BACP 2016:37)*

Despite the good intentions, such blanket descriptions of 'the' culture can veer dangerously close to the kind of racially and religiously loaded denigration of Arabic culture that characterises a particular strain of contemporary Northern European racism; this is a perspective keen to use a particular vision of gender equity of comparative recent emergence in its own culture as a stick to beat the 'backward' Arabs with.

This contemporary use of the 'culture concept' raises the issue in a particular manner directed towards particular contemporary ends. The current explosion of interest in cultural difference is expressive of a particular vision of liberal multicultural governance, which seeks not only to use the 'culture concept' to raise attention to issues and dynamics that were perhaps previously all too often overlooked but also to enforce the adoption of a perspective based on its premises through mechanisms such as training and regulatory regimes. The idea of 'culture' becomes a way of making tangible certain kinds of intangible or numerically immeasurable differences in order for those tasked with managing diverse populations towards an organisational or governmental aim. As Urciuoli (2009:21) observes in her study of 'diversity discourses' in a US liberal arts college, it becomes a means by which the university leadership attempts to secure a particular entrepreneurial style of management that makes different groups responsible for presenting their complex and shifting attitudes towards racial differences in a coherent manner, and thus becomes a constitutive element of 'a neoliberalization of racial markedness, as in the idea of "educating" the community' (ibid).

In this regard, therapy marks just one example of a general trend, noted by Sahlins and many others since the mid-1990s, that the rest of the world is adopting a model of culture that defined anthropology throughout most of the twentieth century just at the moment that anthropologists collectively chose to abandon it. But, as anthropologists have also been increasingly eager to point out in recent decades, this easy-to-use conception of culture comes with a price attached. As the anthropologists Segal and Handler (1995:391) observed back in 1995, for example,

> U.S. multiculturalism often relies upon a hegemonic and essentializing conception of culture. This culture concept . . . represents diversity as a set of discrete and homogeneous units ('cultures'); divides and allots history to living persons on the basis of contemporary identities; conflates culture and race; and obscures the mutual shaping of racial distinctions and class relations. As a result, it limits both criticism of established social institutions and the imagination of alternative social orders.

The very idea of 'having a culture' is one that unites both progressive advocates of identity politics and conservative advocates of unitary nationalism – the idea of a 'culture' as a shared object possessed by a unified group of people is at the heart of both political projects, as Handler (1988) observes in his earlier work, detailing the process that he describes as the 'objectification of culture'. The potential problems of this are described by May (2003:202) when he observes that

> the problems of cultural essentialism and the reification of group-based identities . . . mobilised so effectively by racist proponents, also continue ironically to haunt much multicultural theory and practice. This is particularly evident in multicultural education where the regular invocation of 'cultural difference' often presents culture as *sui generis* (Hoffman 1996). In the process, ethnicity is elided with culture and both come to be treated as 'bounded cultural objects', to borrow a phrase from Richard Handler (1988), which are seen to attach unproblematically to (most usually) ethnic minority students.

A global psychotherapy

As psychotherapy spreads globally, the assumption that it is a Western practice sustained by 'individualism' will become increasingly difficult to sustain as a target of critique. In a group discussion that I conducted with final year psychotherapy students in Bangalore at the end of 2016, most of the group spontaneously advanced the position that they were at the forefront of a wave that promoted 'individualism' that acted in contrast to what they described as 'traditional Indian culture'. The group was wholeheartedly enthusiastic about their role in this change. For them, 'traditional Indian culture', in this context at least, stood for misogyny, caste discrimination and, most crucially, a lack of control over one's own life choices. Individualism and culture were opposed in this framing, as in others that have been discussed in this chapter, but the idea of 'adapting' themselves or clients to the culture, as they had discursively framed it for the purpose of this particular conversation, was not on the agenda. As one of them told me, 'we are in the vanguard of changing the culture'. However, the story does not end there, for as the discussion continued, doubts began to be raised about the word 'individualism'. Did it really sum up what they wanted to get across to me? Some began to fear that it implied a rejection of relations and began to suggest instead that what they stood for was a 'differentiation' from 'traditional' relations that would allow them to enter into more real and fulfilling relations with others: relations that they went on to describe as the basis for making themselves and their future clients into different kinds of people.

'Individualism' never meant for these students an autonomous bounded bogey-man waiting to be imposed upon them by Western influences, including psychotherapeutic theory. Rather, it always meant an attempt to re-shape particular kinds of relations in order to re-shape the culture (not to reject culture or to adapt to an objectified fetish of 'the' culture) and in so doing to re-shape themselves as persons in relation with others (not to become individuals outside of relations). In the course of the conversation, it became clear to them that the very term might carry the connotation of a 'Western individualism', so they differentiated it from that with the term 'differentiating' from traditional relations. At first, 'individualism' carried that connotation for them, and then as the conversation continued, it began to carry a different connotation that enabled them to more accurately define their own sensibilities in contrast to it. This process of differentiating meanings in the shifting contexts of different conversations is the precisely the process of how meaning is made intersubjectively and demonstrates the importance of paying attention to the particular shifting differentiations and meanings that are made by particular words in particular contexts. This is a realisation that should be fundamentally shared as a basic tenet of practice between anthropologists and psychotherapists, yet it is in danger of being overlooked in the rush towards textbook-derived understandings of other people's 'cultures'. If this is the case for a group discussion of therapy students, then it will equally well be the case for our clients as well in their discussion of work, family, friends, 'culture' and their own 'individuality', whether rejected or aspired to in a particular moment. It should remind us that a sensitive appreciation of what terms like 'individual' or 'culture' mean in a particular conversational context will help us to be aware of the contradictory ways in which validating the 'culture' against 'individualism' might be experienced. In particular it might remind us that such a rhetorical move might be felt as being equally or even more oppressive by those we seek to take more seriously through the addition of 'culture' to therapy than the problem of 'individualism' being imposed upon those who possess a different 'culture'. The Bangalore students were aware that they were negatively characterised as 'Western individualists' by those who saw them as part of a wave of cultural change threatening traditional patterns of obligation and obedience. Defending the 'culture' against 'individualism' can carry as much danger to those whom we might easily characterise as coming from 'other' cultural backgrounds as the assumption of a wave of insensitive Western individualism destroying cultural difference.

Conclusion

Rather than assuming that 'culture' is something outside of therapy to be incorporated as an external object, we can perhaps begin by looking at what work is done by its separation and consequent re-incorporation and addition by some to the therapeutic process. What is potentially positive in its addition is that it can address lacunae that might have led therapists to pathologise behaviour that seemed bizarre or maladaptive from the therapist's perspective, but inevitable or expressive of a healthy state of self in relation to others for those with a different (cultural) sense of the appropriate limits and degrees of relational obligation. If claims to 'individuality' are always at heart 'relational', in different regards and to differing degrees, then it is of course possible that the kinds of relations that one acknowledges as a part of the constitution of a healthy individualism can vary across historical epochs or 'cultures' (however defined); as of course they can between family members, or the same individual person at different stages of her life-cycle. 'Culture' can and has been a highly useful heuristic tool in pointing therapists towards aspects of that ongoing dynamic, for example, where otherwise they might have seen unhealthy degrees of dependence. But just as it is the case that an unquestioned prioritisation of the 'individual' self might lead us to a blindness of wider relational fields (sometimes usefully glossed as 'culture'), it is wise for us to be aware of the potential dangers in overenthusiastically grasping the other end of the conceptual opposition in an attempt to redress the alleged imbalances of the past.

If a focus on an unexamined particular manifestation of 'individuality' carries the danger of pathologising behaviour that might seem perfectly healthy to others, then a focus on 'culture' as the corrective opposition to that focus carries other dangers, not least the normalisation of behaviour that those who we have defined as culturally 'Other' might be tentatively exploring their conflicting feelings regarding. At its worst, it can be a tool as capable of inflicting clumsy and hurtful insensitivity upon a client's attempt to make sense of their own life-world as surely as a 'culture-blind' assumption of a particular kind of individual autonomy can be. In my training, we were repeatedly made aware of the dangers of a 'Western' or 'Eurocentric' bias creating barriers to therapeutic effectiveness. For example, in the article by Khan mentioned earlier, he tells the reader of a friend who 'ended the counseling prematurely because he felt the counselor approached his problems from a Eurocentric perspective' (Khan 2013:21). The opposite danger, that 'cultural' framings might be experienced as oppressive or as an equal barrier to therapeutic effectiveness, was almost never raised. During my training, I was discussing personal therapy with an acquaintance of mine from outside Europe. He described recounting a history of abusive behaviour from relatives in his extended family from an early age. The therapist's response was to ask if that was normal or common 'in your culture'? While my acquaintance said that he was aware that the question was probably well-intentioned, the effect on him was traumatic and led to a breakdown of whatever chance there might have been of a strong therapeutic alliance developing. What he heard when he was asked if this was normal 'in his culture' was 'is this acceptable in your culture' and, as a consequence, 'is it okay that this happened to you?' McLeod (1999:219) is keen on occasion to add caveats to his argument that the therapist's job is to 'strengthen the culture', to the effect that he is 'not arguing that counseling promotes conformity to prevailing social rules, norms and values' – although he immediately qualifies this qualification by adding, 'to some extent it must do'. But it is easy to see in a therapeutic encounter how such a 'cultural sensitivity' could lead in the direction of the therapist crushing the first tender steps towards an expression of feelings and thoughts that the client is exploring as her own for the first time. We can compare this perhaps with Rogers' views on the subject, as an earlier writer to whom McLeod is consciously setting up his position in opposition. Rogers (1961:105–106) describes the self-actualised person arising from person-centred therapy as someone who, when his

> awareness of experience . . . is most fully operating, then he is to be trusted, his behavior is constructive. It is not always conventional. It will not always be conforming. It will be individualized. But it will also be socialized.

As anthropologists have increasingly argued since the mid-1970s, 'culture' is not a thing out there in the world but rather a concept or idea designed to make potentially unfamiliar aspects of the ever-evolving mess of social life comprehensible and manageable. As such, it is not a thing, but a shorthand for an infinite number of processes, relations and perspectives, designed to bring certain features into focus in order to make them visible, recognise them and manage them. In this regard, it is similar to the Russian socio-linguist Valentin Volosinov's (1986[1929]) observations concerning language: that there is no such thing as *the* English language or Russian language. Every speaker speaks differently from each other, and differently from how they have spoken previously in different contexts. They do not do this in a vacuum, as 'autonomous individuals', but in relation to others who are themselves subtly changing both their own use of language and the unspoken rules and norms of the language in interaction with them. This is not to say that the idea of the English language or a system of English grammar is not useful. Such generalising concepts are essential as 'translation devices', enabling speakers of Russian to get to grips with the meanings embedded in English speakers' discourse. But the English grammar in a textbook is never precisely the same as any speaker actually uses it in real life, and Volosinov's point is that *this* 'English language' as an object does not actually exist outside of the translator's necessary desire to codify it for those who need such a device. While this is often a necessary step for understanding elements of languages, the danger according to Volosinov is that linguists can make the concept that they have created to aid the study of languages, itself into the object of study, a position that he cautions against as one of 'abstract formalism'.

The same can be said for 'culture'. It is a concept designed to make aspects of shared experience understandable to someone who is currently outside of that shared experience. And to that extent, it can be immensely useful. In my own experience, there have been a number of occasions that it has aided my understanding of a client and the client's ability to feel that they are able to communicate aspects of their experience that they fear will be unfamiliar or incomprehensible to me. And in all of those cases, it has been when the client themselves have advanced the concept, in some variety of 'in my culture', to point me towards aspects of a wider social context beyond immediate family or close personal relations that *they* have felt *in that moment* would be useful to me for understanding why they or others behaved or felt in a particular manner. But as Volosinov would also observe, like any other word, its meaning changes from conversational context to context – what the same speaker is attempting to point to using the word in a conversation with her therapist may not be the same thing as she is attempting to highlight in a conversation with her father or her social worker. Being sensitive to the meaning of a client's 'culture', as much as anything, relies upon a sensitivity to what she might be trying to communicate with the concept in a particular moment more than it does on presuming that she has a culture, separate from herself, that the therapist can acquire expert knowledge of from lectures, textbooks or research papers. Like terms such as 'transference', 'culture' is a double-edged sword for both client and therapist alike – potentially pointing towards or away from the reality and discomfort of feelings that emerge in the encounter. 'Culture' does not always have to be, as in Snyder's description, a means by which the client avoids talking about herself, but can be a means by which she reveals aspects of herself that might otherwise be difficult to articulate to someone who does not share aspects of her experience. But we should be wary of simply dismissing Snyder's position as the defensive posture of one attached to an old-fashioned and out-dated psychological universalism.

Working as a trainee therapist at a university counselling service in the UK, I was struck by how often an anxiety about connectivity to social media was raised by clients. The problem was typically raised as one in which the client wished to remove themselves from being ever-available on social media via their phones, but fearing that even temporary removal would be interpreted by others as an act of hostility, rejection or aggression. And this was a problem that was often relayed to me as 'part of the culture nowadays'. In the context of our therapeutic conversations, these young adults were using the culture concept to translate something of their own shared experience with others such as themselves to someone of an older generation that they suspected might not share the experience or know what it felt like to be entangled in it. In this context, it served to normalise a state of affairs that might seem abnormal to me, but in a manner that seemed to work in precisely the opposite way from my acquaintance's description of his therapist's clumsy introduction of 'culture' in his therapy; in this case, it enabled them to express a part of their own experience that they knew that there was a good chance that I would not intuitively grasp as 'normal'.

However, while all the uses of 'culture' to explain this state of affairs to me did seem to share this feature, they were nuanced in terms of how I experienced different clients making use of it. Some clients described how difficult it was to take control of social media connectivity and carve out a space for themselves where they were free of its demands for particular periods. Others described it as 'impossible' to do so, because of 'the culture'. The examples of the other students who had resisted social pressure to disconnect for periods demonstrated that the 'culture' was not forcing all young people to remain connected to Instagram 24/7, but in these other cases reference to the 'culture' became *among other things* a means by which these clients sought to avoid exploring the personally specific reasons why they felt unable to do so. In these cases, 'culture' acted both as a means by which the client made available to me aspects of her own experience that she feared I might have otherwise found hard to grasp *and* as a distancing mechanism by which the client avoided exploring aspects of her own person, as Snyder suggests might be the case. There is no necessary opposition between the two – indeed, they might both be present in the very same moment.

This kind of virtual connectivity is often imagined by members of an older generation as being an example of and means by which a younger generation asserts its 'individual' freedom from its elders. I have heard it described as such by other therapists in the UK, and on my trip to Bangalore, it was described as a means by which young people assert their individual freedom from traditional culture by a psychologist responsible for running therapy training at the university that I was visiting. This conversation instantly took me back to my clients in the UK a couple of years earlier, and what struck me was that for them, internet connectivity often felt like something that tied them into a 'culture' that they felt threatened their individual freedom and autonomy. What is brought into being as the 'culture' when viewed from one perspective can seem radically different from the 'culture' that is brought into being when viewed from another, as can the nature of the 'individual' that is either threatened or enabled by it. And what this illustrates is that the skills traditionally encouraged by both anthropological fieldwork and therapeutic encounters of carefully listening to the nuances of words and the work that they do in separating out aspects of lived experience remain central.

There is some fleeting awareness of this potential understanding of the use of 'culture' as a performative linguistic act through which persons re-shape themselves in the contemporary literature. For example, in the BACP research overview of diversity issues mentioned above, there is a fascinating mention of research that demonstrates the ways in which people who become deaf later in life

> tend to perceive hearing loss either as a disability, or as a medical condition, rather than a cultural experience, and they must therefore come to terms with, or adjust to, a new self-concept or identity. . . . As such, they experienced emotional turmoil when negotiating issues of identity and belongingness.
>
> *(BACP 2016:23)*

What this might tell us is that whether something is a 'cultural' factor or not is not written in stone, but that rather the very separation of aspects of one's experience into 'culture' and 'other' factors is itself a powerful part of the processes by which selves are made and remade. An increased sensitivity to the work that 'culture' does in these instances can be invaluable therapeutically. But rather than this insight being the basis for further discussion of the work of culture in this regard, it is mentioned in passing, and the predominant framing of 'culture' as the objective property of bounded groups that the therapist needs to educate herself on outside of the therapeutic encounter remains pre-eminent.

And if it is true that 'culture' can simultaneously work as a mechanism that can both bring aspects of lived experience to the foreground and obscure them for the client, then is this not potentially the case for the therapist as well? Is it not the case that 'culture' could on some occasions act as means for the therapist to avoid dealing with the person in front of her, of partially objectifying her in order to avoid dealing with the uncomfortable feelings that her story or feeling might evoke? Could it not, all too easily, become a means of expert manipulation of difficult and alien material, that makes it easier to handle by virtue of being placed in that box? Is it not the case that on occasion it is not only the client but the therapist who might prefer to talk about 'culture' than to talk about or look into herself? The current BACP Ethical Framework seems to explicitly encourage this tendency. Good Practice Point 22g enjoins members to

> recognise when our knowledge of key aspects of our client's background, identity or lifestyle is inadequate and take steps to inform ourselves from other sources where available and appropriate, rather than expecting the client to teach us.
>
> *(BACP 2018b:20)*

But who better to tell us what the client's background, identity, lifestyle (or culture) means to them *in that moment than the client themselves*? The danger that therapists who are genuinely uncomfortable with difference can use such 'expert knowledge' as a means of hiding from the discomfort of an encounter with a client who is struggling with ambiguous feelings about their 'culture' – while publicly performing 'respect' for difference and diversity by placing it in the box marked 'culture' – should be all too apparent. The BACP's Diversity overview document includes the claim that unexplored 'cultural' assumptions can all too easily carry the danger that the, 'the counsellor will consciously, or unconsciously, take the stance of an expert of the client' (BACP 2016:17). Maybe so, but if understanding 'culture' means working with a model of 'culture' as an object that tells us that 'Arabs have rigid gender' or 'South Asians are more religious' that we have learnt from textbooks, then it is precisely that model of 'cultural competence' that increasingly carries a far greater danger than an assumed 'Western individualism' in that regard.

The rise of 'culture' as a factor separate from the processes going on within and between therapist and client in their encounter is increasingly marked in training and practice as well as in theory. In my training, culture was dealt with in a series of separate stand-alone lectures. This always felt inadequate, itself perhaps an inevitable result of this separation of cultural processes into culture and the assumed backdrop of Western individualism that most trainees were assumed to unproblematically adhere to. But given that that separation was the only strategy on hand for taking 'culture' seriously, the only strategy available to address that shortcoming under discussion was to increase the amount of time devoted to lectures and abstract discussion of the subject, at the cost of losing time devoted to development of reflexive skills on therapeutic practice. In this regard, the move towards cultural sensitivity *as it is currently being organised and taught* fits in with a wider agenda of 'professionalisation' pushed by the leadership of organisations such as BACP, in which particular sets of auditable 'skills' or 'competencies' become the benchmark of 'best practice'. When viewed from this perspective, the separation out of culture into an object that the practitioner demonstrates 'expert' knowledge of having learnt becomes an instance of the kind of use of 'culture' as a technique of neoliberal educational governance as described by Urciuoli for liberal education more generally.

Developing a sensibility for the shifting meanings and importance of 'cultural' factors requires a development of the kind of personal qualities that anthropology and psychotherapy training have often valued and sought to nurture. If 'culture' is a concept in the therapist's mind during therapy or reflection upon it, then surely, like other such concepts, a good starting point is to ask what is it doing in *this* particular conversational or reflective context? What does framing this particular part of the interaction or description as 'culture' do from the client's point of view? Perhaps most crucially, what does framing it as 'culture' do for *me* as the therapist in this moment? What happens when I separate out aspects of the experience and categorise those as 'culture'? Is it in this moment a bridge to greater understanding? Or in this moment might it be operating as a distancing mechanism that objectifies 'culture', and in so doing potentially partially objectifies the person that I frame as possessing it in order to aid my understanding?

It is not hard to see how 'culture' can potentially do both of these things; in order to be alive to the potential pros and cons of its use in shifting contexts, we have to be aware emotionally of the work that it is doing for *us* in any particular moment. Otherwise it runs the risk of becoming another potentially useful tool that can unintentionally pathologise the patient, such as 'transference'. *That* understanding cannot be achieved from text-book or power-point summaries of cultural difference but fundamentally relies upon the continued development of a self-awareness and the cultivation of a disposition as a person who is capable of listening and being surprised by what the client says and one's own responses to it. If this is what is meant by arguing that 'half a day on "diversity issues" isn't going to do it', then it is hard to disagree. The development of a sensitivity to one's own (cultural) blind spots, including the role of framing some issues to oneself as cultural and some as not, will not be achieved in half a day but has to be part of the wider and longer term development of a therapeutic self. If what is meant, however, is that the current half day power-point display on diversity and different cultures is expanded into a week at the continuing cost to the spaces that encourage the potential development of that awareness of shifting meaning in relation with clients, then it is a claim with the capacity to do as much harm as good.

References

BACP. (2016). *Good Practice in Action 056: Research Overview of Equality, Diversity and Inclusion in the Counselling Professions*. Lutterworth: BACP.

BACP. (2018a). *Counsellor/Psychotherapist Accreditation Scheme Application Pack*. Lutterworth: BACP.

BACP. (2018b). *Ethical Framework for the Counselling Professions*. Lutterworth: BACP.

Benedict, R. (1934). *Patterns of Culture*. New York: Houghton Mifflin Company.

Berne, E. (1975). *What Do You Say after You Say Hello?* London: Corgi.

Cameron, R. (2017). Culture and Context. *Therapy Today*. 28(1):30–33.

Crawford, M. (2017). *Personal Correspondence*. 15.05.2017.

Crawford, M., Lavanya, T., Farquharson, L., Palmer, L., Hancock, E., Bassett, P., Clarke, H. and Parry, G. (2016). Patient Experience of Negative Effects of Psychological Treatment: Results of a National Survey. *The British Journal of Psychiatry*. 208:260–265.

d'Ardenne, P. and Mahtani, A. (1999). *Transcultural Counselling in Action*. London: Sage.

Dhillon, K. and Ubhi, M. (2006). Acculturation and Ethnic Identity in Marginal Immigrant South Asian Men in Britain: A Psychotherapeutic Perspective. *Counselling and Psychotherapy Research*. 3(1):42–48.

Douglas, M. and Isherwood, B. (1979). *The World of Goods: Towards an Anthropology of Consumption*. New York. Norton. Cited in Dhillon, K. and Ubhi, M. (2006). Acculturation and Ethnic Identity in Marginal Immigrant South Asian Men in Britain: A Psychotherapeutic Perspective. *Counselling and Psychotherapy Research*. 3(1):42–48.

Erikson, E. (1977[1951]). *Childhood and Society*. London: Triad/Paladin Books.

Freud, S. (1991[1905]). Three Essays on the Theory of Sexuality. In S. Freud. *On Sexuality: Three Essays on the Theory of Sexuality and Other Works*. London: Penguin.

Handler, R. (1988). *Nationalism and the Politics of Culture in Quebec*. Madison: University of Wisconsin Press.

Hoffman, D. (1996). Culture and Self in Multicultural Education: Reflections on Discourse, Text and Practice. *American Educational Research Journal*. 33:545–569.

Jackson, C. (2016). Editorial: Learning from our Mistakes. *Therapy Today*. 27(3):3.

Jenkins, P. (2011). Issues of Race and Culture in Counselling. *Course Handout*. Manchester: University of Manchester.

Khan, A. (2013). How I Became a Therapist. *Therapy Today*. 24(8):21.

Lloyd, K. (2014). *Counsellor/Psychotherapist Accreditation Scheme: Criterion 9: Practice and Supervision*. Available at www.bacp.co.uk/media/1520/bacp-individual-accreditation-application-guide-criterion-9.pdf. Accessed 30.08.2018.

Malinowski, B. (1927). *Sex and Repression in Savage Society*. London: Kegan Paul/Trench, Trubner and Co. Ltd.

May, S. (2003). Critical Multiculturalism. *Counterpoints*. 168:199–212.

McLeod, J. (1999). Counselling as a Social Process. *Counselling*. 10(3):217–222.

McLeod, J. (2003) *An Introduction to Counselling*. Philadelphia: Open University Press.

Miller, A. (1990[1979]). *The Drama of the Gifted Child: The Search for the True Self*. New York: Basic Books.

Rogers, C. (1951). *Client-Centered Therapy*. London: Constable.

Rogers, C. (1961). *On Becoming a Person: A Therapist's View of Psychotherapy*. London: Constable.

Segal, D. and Handler, R. (1995). U.S. Multiculturalism and the Concept of Culture. *Identities*. 1(4):391–407.

Snyder, E. (2014). The Shibboleth of Cross-Cultural Issues in Psychoanalytic Treatment. Pp. 91–98. In D. Scharff and S. Varvin (eds.) *Psychoanalysis in China*. London: Karnac Books.

Urciuoli, B. (2009). Talking/Not Talking about Race: The Enregisterments of 'Culture' in Higher Education Discourse. *Journal of Linguistic Anthropology*. 19(1):21–39.

Volosinov, V. (1986[1929]). *Marxism and the Philosophy of Language*. Cambridge: Harvard University Press.

5

HISTORY IN THE PSYCHE, PARTICLES IN THE SELF

The case of Z

Karen Seeley

History in the psyche

There is a gathering view that academic disciplines have outlived their usefulness. Psychoanalysis and anthropology emerged in the midst of an era when the delineation of separate fields – each with its own language, methods, and aims – was thought to spur the production of knowledge. More than a century later, some scholars no longer believe that their discipline possesses privileged access to the truth. In light of "realities and problems which are ever more global, transnational, multidimensional, transversal, polydisciplinary and planetary" (Morin, 2001:29), they see the segregation of disciplines, and of intellectual communities, as barriers to inquiry, and they seek to generate knowledge by cutting across academic domains.

Further, as French psychoanalyst Sacha Nacht observed, disciplinary boundaries are artificial. Nacht (cited in Lacan, 1996:237) stated that "it should not be forgotten that the division into embryology, physiology, psychology, sociology and clinical medicine does not exist in nature." His claim equally applies to the division between anthropology and psychoanalysis. And yet, contemporary psychoanalysts and cultural anthropologists are likely to assert that their fields have long been divorced on the grounds of irreconcilable differences. To be sure, these two disciplines vary in many respects; however, the approaches developed by their founders, Franz Boas and Sigmund Freud, have important similarities. Both approaches are centered on listening to people talk. Both search for themes and patterns that are outside respondents' awareness. Both are interested in deep meaning, and in the origins of present phenomena. Their shared commitments to observation and language, and to history, pattern, and symbol, remain essential to their fields. In addition, the founder of each field created a body of work that transcended his discipline's boundaries. Freud's case studies of individual patients speak volumes about a society and an era; Boas's ethnographies of cultures provide us with complex portraits of human behavior and mind.

Despite apparent intersections in their interests and approaches, disciplinary boundaries were drawn. Put simply, anthropologists came to investigate the external world of culture, while psychoanalysts took as their domain the internal world of the mind. This artificial division remains foundational to psychoanalytic theory and practice. Ever since Freud (1896) renounced his seduction hypothesis, having determined that patients' stories of sexual abuse were fantastical rather than real (Masson, 1984), he "tended to close his mind to the significance of environment" (Thompson, 1950:9). Psychoanalysts followed suit, offering accounts of hermetically sealed minds that are exclusively at the mercy of intrapsychic oscillations. Even contemporary analysts who identify as interpersonalists claim that taking the environment into account is tantamount to "forsaking our unique and powerful perspective" (Kuriloff, 2001:673). Instead of seeing the mind and the worlds it inhabits as mutually constitutive (Shweder, 1991), many continue to isolate the mind from all context – from culture and community, politics and history – and insist on the absolute primacy of the unconscious and the psychic interior.

For psychoanalysts and psychotherapists, the absence of cultural perspectives is not only a theoretical question but also an urgent practical matter. This absence constricts the work of analytic dyads that are international, intercultural, and interracial – in which it is more and more likely that patients as well as analysts are culturally, linguistically, and racially diverse. Moreover, it inhibits analytic reflection on the processes by which ostensibly exterior contexts and events, including individuals' political and cultural histories, make their marks on the self.

How might we reconcile a psychoanalysis, whose head is entirely in the head, with an anthropology, whose feet are planted firmly on the ground? This chapter works to undo the unnatural separation between the individual mind and its cultural and political surrounds and to restore their interconnections. While no single historical moment or theoretical statement can be held solely responsible for psychoanalysis's dismissal of the social worlds its patients inhabit, I consider a particular period in which this dismissal gathered force. In the first part of this chapter, I examine the fortification of boundaries between interior and exterior worlds in psychoanalytic theory and practice in the United States during World War II and the postwar. In the second part of this chapter, I discuss my work with a patient in my private practice, situating her subjectivity, emotional states, and plural senses of self in her history of migration, and in her family's traumatic history of political violence, displacement, and loss.

According to Bettelheim (1990), the decline of the Habsburg Empire, which once had extended across the globe, created circumstances that were favorable to the creation of psychoanalysis. At the Empire's peak, Vienna was famed for its cosmopolitanism, for its sciences and its arts, and for its political and economic clout. But as the Empire lost territory and power, and as social conditions grew chaotic, frightened citizens turned inward, shielding their eyes from the collapse of their world. In Bettelheim's view, the empire's calamitous decline gave rise to a theory of mind that privileged the intrapsychic, while rendering exterior worlds insignificant. Freud's new theory of psychoanalysis excised the psyche from its contexts, negating the very surroundings that had caused it so much harm.

Psychoanalysis's emphasis on the interior world of a decontextualized subject served additional purposes. For one, it provided its founder with cover for his stigmatized social identities as an immigrant and a Jew. In Vienna, Eastern European immigrants like Sigmund Freud and his family were treated with special disdain. The medical textbooks of Freud's era stated that Jews were mentally defective, and prone to severe psychiatric illness (Gilman, 1993). Such prejudices cast doubt on Freud's work as a scientist and slowed his professional advancement. In response to his hostile surroundings, Freud created a theory of a unitary mind. This theory was a statement of human equality; it was an elaborate refutation of the virulent anti-Semitism that marked him as diseased and intellectually deficient. According to Freud, persons' acquired characteristics – whether religious and cultural affiliations or histories of immigration – affected neither the contents nor the workings of their mental life. Rather, every mind was governed by the same biological drives, and by the operations of identical psychic structures.

The disavowal of stigmatized identities, and the turning away from social and political worlds that inflicted terror and pain, had been integral to the origins of psychoanalysis. They became its motifs. Before and during World War II, Jewish émigré and refugee psychoanalysts who fled to America to escape Nazi Germany followed Freud's example. Some arrived in America shattered and defeated. They had escaped a genocidal regime that had terrorized, interned, and starved them; murdered their family and friends; ripped them apart from their children; razed their homes and communities; stripped them of their professions; and expelled them from where they were born.

Paradoxically, the influx of analysts from Europe, where millions of people had been exterminated, gave American psychoanalysis a vital shot of life. Upon their arrival in the US, the Europeans presented psychoanalytic institutes with "an astounding collection of analytic talent" (Makari, 2008:461). Yet some Americans feared that the sheer volume of new talent would overwhelm the market. As a result, their welcome was less than wholehearted, and some were more welcomed than others. Viennese analysts who had seen Freud in the flesh, or who claimed a genealogical connection – for example, by having been analyzed by an analyst who had been analyzed by Freud – enjoyed prestige and authority. Europeans quickly rose to power in the American psychoanalytic establishment. By 1961, every official of the New York Psychoanalytic Institute was an immigrant, and half of them were from Vienna (Thompson, 2012).

In spite of their high profile, European analysts kept their personal histories quiet, disavowing debased identities as Holocaust victims and as Jews (Kuriloff,

2014). Indeed, after resettling in the States, they reproduced the patterns that Bettelheim identified as central to the creation of psychoanalysis. In Europe they had been trained to privilege the intrapsychic and to disregard the emotional impacts of exterior events. When their patients began to describe the extreme persecution and brutality they had suffered in Nazi Germany, analysts focused narrowly on their interior world. Turning away from survivors' stories of actual violence and loss, they took shelter in a theory and practice that rigidly enforced the construction of an isolated mind inside a decontextualized subject. Even the political Freudians (Jacoby, 1983:9), who escaped to the States from Berlin and Vienna, turned their backs on the external world. Before coming to America, they had been socialists, Marxists, and activists. For them, psychoanalysis was more than a method of individual treatment; it was equally a project of societal change and political repair. However, once the political Freudians went into exile, they renounced their social commitments in order to better blend into their new nation's conservative fabric. Conforming to the norms of the local analytic community, they took up its apolitical and medicalized forms of practice, adopting a "decultured" psychoanalysis (Jacoby, 1983:6).

And yet for psychoanalysts from Europe, clinical spaces in the States were anything but decultured; rather, in these spaces, they encountered American patients. Analysts thus had to manage the arduous task of treating patients from an alien society while speaking a foreign tongue. Their clinical work with European patients who were refugees, emigres, or Holocaust survivors was even more distressing, as it triggered shattering memories of their personal terror and flight. Struggling to contain their own losses, they policed the classical boundary between patients' interior and exterior worlds. By severing all bonds between them, psychoanalysts tried to ensure that all that they wished to forget, and found too unbearable to remember, was cast out of the clinical frame (Kuriloff, 2014).

But in struggling to quiet their memories and emotions, analysts also silenced their patients. Rather than encouraging patients to say whatever came into their minds, many prohibited them from speaking of how they had been terrorized during the war. In addition, some neglected to examine how patients' constant exposures to organized cruelty and threat were inextricably linked to their current psychic distress. Instead, analysts reduced patients' suffering to intrapsychic conflict, to unconscious wishes and fantasies, and to early childhood injuries. In doing so, they placed patients' histories of political violence and exile, and of cultural destruction and loss, outside the psychoanalytic gaze (Aron & Starr, 2013; Kuriloff, 2014).

Just as European analysts' efforts to suppress their harrowing wartime experiences constricted their clinical practices, they impeded theoretical advancement. Despite analysts' firsthand knowledge of the psyche's vulnerability to unrelenting horror and violence, they turned away from their histories and failed to use their lived experience to enlarge psychoanalytic theory. Rather, they clung to the classical model, constructing interior psychic worlds that were extracted from, and invulnerable to, environmental assaults. By turning theory into "an armor" (Laub cited in Kuriloff, 2014:59), they protected themselves against the brutalities of the Holocaust.

Although these theories served defensive purposes, they masqueraded as doctrine. Psychoanalysts advanced theoretical perspectives that only tacitly gestured at their personal knowledge of atrocity and its psychological effects. Heinz Hartmann escaped Vienna in 1938 – after the Nazis had annexed Austria and categorized his wife and sons as Jews – and resettled in New York City. Yet Hartmann's major work on Ego Psychology proposed a theory of the ego's development within an "average expectable environment" (Hartmann, 1958:51) which was stable and benign, an environment to which infants were biologically adapted, and which they had the capacity to master. He noted only in passing that some environments were neither average nor expectable, so that infants lacked the capacity to master and to survive them. While Hartmann was all too familiar with environments that were unstable and life threatening, he failed to specify their features, their prevalence, and the psychic collapse they wrought. Heinz Kohut, who fled Vienna in 1939, spent a year in a refugee camp in England before ending up in Chicago (Strozier, 2001). Kohut believed that his displacement had split his sense of self into two distinct and irreconcilable pieces. This experience inspired his interest in selves that are unable to achieve cohesion (Quinn, 1984); his concept of the "fragmenting self" refers to the loss of the "sense of the continuity of his self in time and of its cohesiveness in space" (Kohut & Wolf, 1978:418). Although Kohut's personal fragmentation resulted from political persecution and threat – including the explicit threat that his son would be sent to a concentration camp (Strozier, 2001) – his theory of Self Psychology traced such fragmentation solely to early self-object failures. Margaret Mahler, who fled Vienna in 1938, arrived in Philadelphia the same year. America was so painfully distant from her family and colleagues that "only the Nazis could have sent me there" (Mahler & Stepansky, 1988:94). Mahler recalled her "excruciating farewell" to her mother, where she sat on her mother's lap "and clung to her like a baby" (Mahler & Stepansky, 1988:90). Although the separation from her mother, who later died in Auschwitz, was due to the Nazi occupation of Austria, in Mahler's extensive research on infants' separation and individuation, she theorized separation only as an intrapsychic and physiological process (Mahler, 1967).

The works of these three European analysts are, in essence, "ethnotheories" (Estroff 1993:254) of abnormality and normality, in that they are rooted in highly specific political and social contexts. They are remarkable for what they exclude, and for their authors' skill at cutting the links between severe psychological injuries and the conditions that inflict them. Prince (2009) claims that psychoanalysis is a Holocaust survivor: that having barely outlived a regime that was bent on its destruction, it buried its history of atrocity in order to stay alive. Displaced and refugee European analysts also buried their histories of atrocity, producing models of psychoanalysis that failed to recognize the sources of their wounds. These models were without culture, without calamity, without brutality – they were utterly devoid of every form of exteriority. When patients tried to speak about their wartime histories in treatment, their analysts dismissed such accounts as superficial (Kakar, 1985), and as resistances to exploring deep unconscious conflicts. This "conspiracy of silence" (Danieli, 1984:24) persisted. Several decades later, patients still were prohibited from discussing Holocaust memories in clinical encounters. Additional reasons have been offered to explain this tenacious silencing. Perhaps European analysts' allegiance to Freudian imperatives, including analytic neutrality and anonymity, intensified in exile (Makari, 2008). Perhaps having barely escaped anti-Semitism in Europe, they stifled discussions of the Holocaust to ward off anti-Semitism in America. Perhaps as recent immigrants, they thought it prudent to celebrate the "good war" rather than mourning those who were slaughtered, whether on the battlefield, in concentration camps, or by atomic weapons. Or perhaps in the grip of a "manic defense" (Aron & Starr, 2013:123), they embraced America's triumph, and its enthusiasm for the future, to drown out the agony of the past.

Certainly, analysts of that era lacked a conceptual framework for the psychological havoc that exterior catastrophes wreak on the mind – a framework for their patients' wounds, as well as their own. Because Freud was unable to integrate conceptions of trauma into his metapsychology, trauma became "the black hole in the middle of psychoanalytic theory" (Boulanger, 2002:38). Two seminal works on trauma had little impact on psychoanalysts. Kardiner's (1941) study of the traumatic neuroses of war, which examined the damage combat inflicted on soldiers in World War I, proved of little interest to analysts treating civilians (Young, 1995). Krystal's (1969) groundbreaking volume on the massive psychic trauma of civilians who lived through the Holocaust included Niederland's (1968) psychiatric findings on survivors' prolonged mental suffering. However, this work arrived too late for analysts who practiced during the war and the postwar.

In consequence, émigré and refugee analysts did not realize that traumatic injuries persisted long after the stressor ceased, or that their onset could be delayed. They did not know that traumatic reactions had a stubborn tendency to be elicited and relived. Only later would they learn that such wounds were transmissible from one generation to the next, and from their patients to them (Epstein, 1979; Figley, 1995); that in rare cases where both they and their patients had been scarred by the same events, the chance of emotional contagion multiplied (Seeley, 2008); and that the mixture of such factors might cause them to silence their patients, so as to be protected from "reliving some portion of an unmastered past" (Bergmann, 1982:249).

In 1980, the third edition of psychiatry's Diagnostic and Statistical Manual of Mental Disorders (DSM) (APA, 1980) included the new diagnosis of Post-traumatic Stress Disorder. This diagnostic category, which detailed symptomatic responses to a range of environmental stressors, gained a place in the DSM only after biological psychiatry had supplanted psychoanalysis as the "intellectual core of the field" (Shorter, 2015:65), and only after biological psychiatrists had wrested control of the DSM away from psychoanalysts. While PTSD initially was created to address the particular difficulties of returning Vietnam veterans (Shephard, 2000), it drew upon earlier work by Kardiner (1941) and Krystal (1969). Kardiner's (1941) descriptions of key features of war neuroses, including repetitive, threatening dreams and reenactments of traumatic events, influenced PTSD's diagnostic criteria (Young, 1995). Similarly, Krystal's interest in parallel symptoms across disparate groups subjected to persecution and catastrophe informed the construction of PTSD as a universal, biologically based illness. Congruent with Krystal's work, the authors of the DSM-III designed PTSD as a common framework for both civilian and combat traumas. Previously, these types of trauma had been theorized as separate entities; now they were joined together under one overarching category.

In the contemporary psychoanalytic landscape, which is composed of multiple schools with divergent theoretical perspectives, the endorsement of PTSD, and of other notions of trauma, remains decidedly mixed. While interpersonal and relational analysts embrace them, those who are classically trained do not. Freudian analysts remain especially opposed to ideas of adult onset trauma. In their view, only individuals whose psychic structure had been critically weakened in infancy or childhood are susceptible to sustaining traumatic injuries as adults.

This orthodoxy was apparent after the World Trade Center attack in 2001. Although PTSD had been a recognized diagnosis for twenty-one years, many analysts – with the exception of those who had treated veterans of the Vietnam War or survivors of abuse – either were unfamiliar with it or rejected it out of hand. Like analysts who had practiced during World War II and the postwar, a number of New York City psychoanalysts turned away from the mass catastrophe and refused to acknowledge its psychic impacts. Some analysts silenced their patients, discouraging them from discussing their terrifying experiences on 9/11 and their anxieties about additional attacks. Pushing clinical conversations out of the present and into the past, they located patients' wounds in the intrapsychic world, in early childhood histories, and in unconscious fantasies (Seeley, 2008).

The rapid spread of discourses of trauma has given rise to complaints that the "empire of trauma" (Fassin & Rechtman, 2009) has colonized human experience; that trauma has been medicalized, politicized, and globalized in ways that simultaneously trivialize and overextend it. Certainly, psychological theories of trauma are problematic in many respects. Yet, because they contest psychoanalytic notions of separate interior and exterior worlds while also creating bridges between them, they are critically important to analytic theory and practice. PTSD is one of the few psychiatric disorders that cannot be diagnosed without a distinct external stressor. It thus insists that events and conditions that occur in the exterior world profoundly affect the mind; indeed, traumatic wounds are nothing less than the harm the world does to the mind. Theories of trauma force our attention to the ties that bind mental suffering to environmental and historical experience. They authorize explorations of the psychological damage inflicted by political persecution and war, by oppression and institutionalized racism, and by mass disasters and cultural displacement. Rather than conceptualizing analytic patients as decontextualized containers of rigid psychic structures, these theories restore them to the status of whole subjects who are culturally, politically, and historically positioned. Moreover, although psychoanalysis theorizes its subjects as "energetically and affectively self-contained" (Brennan, 2004:2), notions of trauma conceptualize psychic pain not only as individual, but as intersubjective and communal, and as traversing social fields. The concept of intergenerational trauma, which I discuss in the case below, speaks to transpersonal flows of emotion, and of ruptured mental states, in contexts of collective disaster and violence. Abraham (1987/1994) portrays this as a transgenerational haunting, where children unknowingly inherit their parents' unspeakable secrets and calamitous experiences.

The recent emphasis on trauma has brought the belated recognition that psychoanalysis itself has been profoundly impacted by catastrophic circumstances, including mass murder, cultural destruction, and diaspora. This recognition redirects analytic attention to the sorts of experience it has resolutely ignored, and which involve all forms of atrocity, dislocation, disaster, and marginalization. Theories of trauma thus offer psychoanalysts the opportunity to speak to varieties of human experience that, over the course of its history, it has denied and disavowed (Aron & Starr, 2013).

Particles in the self: the case of Z

In the remainder of this chapter, I describe my clinical work with Z. In the discussion that follows, I seek to reestablish the connectedness between the individual mind and its sociocultural and political worlds. Behrouzan (2016:120) claims that "in order to 'be' in present and future spaces, one has to work through pasts that are simultaneously far and near." Z confronted a different task. In order for her to "be" in both the present and the future, she had to work through her individual past, as well as the pasts of her family. Thus, in our work together, I rejected an exclusive focus on Z's interior life. Instead, I grounded her subjectivity in her history of dislocation and in her family's history of political violence and loss. Here, I consider the various ways that the multiple pasts Z's family bequeathed her caused her to experience her self as a collection of disintegrated particles.

In our initial session, Z described herself as depressed. Given her social withdrawal, lack of pleasure, and overriding sadness, she met the diagnostic criteria for depression. In my view, however, her depression was less a disorder of molecules and chemicals than one of politics and history; it was a "cultural and social phenomenon rather than a medical disease" (Cvetkovich, 2012:1). Accordingly, it was essential to attend to the social and political events that had caused the displacements of Z and her family and had shattered her sense of self. In the course of our work together, I tried to grasp the flows of feeling and perception, injury and experience, which were in constant circulation between Z's ostensibly separate internal and external worlds.

When I first met with Z four years ago, she was a college student in her early 20s. She complained of feeling lonely, unhappy, and hopeless; she lived her life in a state of disconnection from everything around her, "just going through the motions." She experienced no pleasure, and she saw "no point in living." She was extremely worried about losing her mother – and then, she said, "I will have nothing." Although Z was ambivalent about being in therapy, she wanted to sort things out for herself, away from the complex force fields of her extended family.

Z told me that when she was 8, she and her family had migrated to the US from Iran, to escape the lengthy aftermath of violent political upheaval. They arrived shortly after 9/11. When Z's mother told her they were going to America, Z imagined it as a large hotel. Upon her arrival it hit her; nearly everything she had ever known was gone. She couldn't decode the language; she couldn't decipher the cultural codes. Z quickly lost her footing, and felt increasingly out of out of place as an immigrant, an Iranian, and a Muslim. For the first several months in her American school, she refused to speak.

Z began to learn English and to adjust to her new environment. But as she did so, she felt her world split apart, and her sense of self fall into pieces. At the time of our first meeting, Z experienced her life as a series of isolated moments, without connective tissue between them. She did not feel that she had a core self, or a cohesive self, or a self that was authentic; only a self that was broken, and had fractured into particles. She tried to control this bedlam of fragments by frantically rearranging them for each specific interaction, so as not be revealed as a "poor, incompetent immigrant." As she moved from one setting to the next – from home, to school, to work, to class, and in and out of every encounter – she altered her self to fit the immediate context, while simultaneously keeping the bits of her self separate and apart.

Z was terrified of uniting the pieces of her self, and she panicked in situations where more than one of them might emerge. She found it equally frightening to experience only one of them. Then Z feared she had lost the others, and none of them, by itself, made her feel that she was whole. But at times the dissimilar parts of herself scolded each other and argued, until she no longer knew which was real, and which one to believe. I encouraged her to bring these various pieces to our sessions, including the more Americanized ones that her family did not acknowledge.

Z often spoke of her mother's extended family, who had migrated to the US around the same time she had arrived. I asked her to draw a family tree so I could get to know her relatives. She drew an elaborate diagram with each member of her family encased in an isolated, self-contained bubble; all were located at varying distances from her personal, self-contained bubble. The diagram resembled the solar system with planets in separate orbits, and as long as they stayed in their orbits, she felt a sense of control.

The colleague who gave Z my name had described me as an anthropologist. Although I am not certain how this affected my work with Z, she may have felt encouraged to foreground the story of her migration, and her family's complex history of dislocation and loss. Moreover, once I realized the depths of the splits in Z's sense of self, I thought it might be useful to characterize her as bicultural. To be sure, she lacked the neat division of experience that this term implies. And yet the term proved fruitful, as it opened up discussions about Z's radical shifts in self from one context to the next. It let us frame these shifts as efforts to adapt to the disparate social worlds in which she had come to reside, and let us focus her reflections on how her cultural and political histories differed from those of her relatives. This term spoke to her lack of cohesion, and to possibilities of integration; it also helped diminish Z's anxiety that she might fall apart.

Z's extended family offered an oasis of support. Yet to be close to them was to be swallowed by their history of trauma. Unlike incidents of displacement where "the past is all of a sudden on one side of a divide, the present on the other" (Hoffman, 1999:46), Z's family remained in the grip of a past that irrupted their present. Though distant in time and space from the political violence they suffered, they still felt under siege.

Z's relatives never discussed their traumatic past with her, but they showed her their misery and pain. She came to know "the vertiginous black hole of the unmentionable years" (Fresco, 1984:418). They tutored her in their worldview. The world is a dangerous place. It is full of crisis and hardship. The government wants to hurt us. No one can be trusted. Thus, Z inherited her uncle's regret for making the choices that ruined his life; she inherited her aunt's grief at losing the people she used to know; she inherited her mother's conviction that the worst would surely happen. Z did not permit herself to feel pleasure, or to realize what she'd gained, for fear of becoming too weak to survive life's inevitable catastrophes. She was certain that, like her family, she would be "stuck in this immigrant place," trapped in a social position that would ensure exclusion and failure.

Could Z's life be anything other than precarity, fracture, and loss? As she began to grasp the nature of the family pasts that she carried, she realized their cost to her sense of cohesion and belonging. Yet she worried what would happen if she were to give them up. Her family's sadness bound them together. If she drew away from their pasts, she might lose her connection to them, and to the place that they had lost. So she continued to be haunted by a past that wasn't hers, and to carry memories that she couldn't remember, of a life that she never had lived.

Z's feelings of inferiority and marginality, and of breaking into pieces, did not belong to her alone. After the second wave of the Iranian diaspora, which lasted from 1979 to 2001, more than 330,000 Persians resettled in the States. Many had been victims of political persecution (PAAIA, 2014). In the wake of political ruptures, where violence and dislocation injure entire communities, some societies foster programs to work through the damage together (Hutchison & Bleiker, 2008). Behrouzan (2016) describes collective, grass roots projects to repair the psychological harm caused by shared historical trauma in Iran. She considers a generation of Iranians who were children at the time of the war between Iran and Iraq, which lasted from 1980 to 1988 and killed over a million people. Nearly thirty years later, members of this generation gather together on social media to assess the remains of their childhood, and to fill in the holes in their lives. On countless blogs and websites, they recall the sights and sounds and sensations that assaulted them during the war. By turning the Internet into an archive of visceral and emotional memory, and into a space of collective mourning, they have created a common language for the flood of events and feelings they had not comprehended as children.

While such communal repair may be critical in instances of collective trauma, Z did not know anyone whose story mirrored her own, nor was she part of a community of shared remembrance and mourning. She had no public culture that gave her history language and meaning, or that helped her refashion her past. Displaced in time as well as in space, stuck in her past as well as her family's, she was unable to write a new narrative that encompassed the possibilities of historical movement and change.

But slowly, Z began to feel better. Life was no longer such a chore. One day, she allowed herself to stop her fevered rush from place to place, and from one piece of her self to another, and to have a cup of coffee. She was doing well in college, where she felt stimulated and happy. She considered the possibility that she might no longer be at the mercy of an inescapable fate; that in contrast to her family, her future was somewhat open. After spending a semester abroad, Z felt less defined by her family's history. She began to refer to her "two sides" – the Iranian side and the American side – without the splintering feeling that she had to choose between them. She began to link the past to the present, and to carefully weave together the fragments of her self.

However, after the terrorist attacks in Paris in November of 2015, Z's injuries reopened, and her sense of self fractured again. As anti-Muslim rhetoric escalated in the US, Z developed a heightened sense of being Muslim and Iranian. If Z previously had suffered at from being culturally unintelligible (Beltsiou, 2016), suddenly she was all too legible. She thought that other students were staring at her in class. When her employer asked her if she was a Muslim, she grew afraid that he would fire her. Reliving personal and family histories of dislocation and marginalization, Z's anxieties overcame her. She feared that she would be deported, or sent to an internment camp. She worried that if she traveled abroad, US customs officials would block her from reentering the States.

Similarly, when Z decided to visit Iran for the first time in many years, her sense of self swung wildly from one pole to the other. At first, her sense of herself as an American obscured all other identities. What if upon arriving the airport, border police identified her as an enemy of the state and threw her out of the country? What if she were walking down an avenue in Tehran and Iranian policemen arrested her and sent her to jail? Z again experienced herself as dangerous and unwanted, and felt destined to live a life defined by banishment and loss. But at the same time, Z grew worried that she would become so attached to Iran that she would decide to stay. In doing so, however, she would re-fracture the sense of self she had painstakingly put together. Indeed, the more Z came to feel like an insider in Iran, the more she stood to lose her entire American life.

After Z returned from Iran, she felt as if her Iranian and American sides again had coalesced. But her newfound sense of cohesion proved to be short-lived. During the 2016 presidential campaign, her self again fell into pieces. Bombarded by campaign speeches urging the deportation of immigrants and spewing anti-Muslim rhetoric, Z re-experienced herself as a threatening outsider. She dreaded sitting next to white passengers on the subway; she was sure they regarded her with suspicion. She described a recent dream in which a group of men were wearing pointed white hoods.

I regarded Z's growing alarm as a rational response to an environment of genuine threat. When Z previously had voiced anxieties about her security and place in America, I had interpreted them through the lens of her losses and uprooting, and of her family's traumatic history. But given the altered political landscape, I no longer viewed Z's terror as a reliving of prior suffering, nor did I reduce it to intrusions of memory and affect due to intergenerational trauma.

This shift in my perspective caused me to question my ability to grasp Z's subjectivity. There is no doubt that my secure status as a white American had caused me to misjudge her precarious social position. Since her arrival in America, Z had been subjected to hostile messages about immigrants – and especially, about Muslim immigrants from Iran – that were less audible to me. The less I heard such messages, the more I attributed her fears about her place in American society to her past and the pasts of her family, rather than to present, pervasive, and virulent anti-immigrant currents.

Many times in our work together, Z had seemed unmoored. Utterly lacking in the hope that she might belong in America, she thought that our sessions were pointless. I too lost heart at times, but I believed that she possessed talents and opportunities that neither her personal and family histories, nor the existing political climate, could entirely outweigh. Although I was well aware that trauma casts a long shadow, I wished to lead her out of it. While fully acknowledging the obstacles in her way, I offered a path forward, and a vision of repair, that Z had not imagined.

And yet it is entirely possible that because I could not fully grasp the catastrophic histories that Z carried, and the social realities that she inhabited, my hopes for her were misplaced. It is possible that I failed to see that her traumatic view of the world was more accurate, more adaptive, and more emotionally resonant than my certainty that she would flourish and claim her place in society.

Conclusion

Some analysts believe that in order to do their work effectively, they must totally immerse themselves in their patients' subjectivities. This approach poses a serious challenge; if analysts are pulled too far into patients' subjectivities, they may have trouble reclaiming their own (Seeley, 2008). But clinical treatments that are intercultural, interracial, and multinational pose a different sort of challenge. As Mitchell (1993:60) noted, "everything that the analyst knows about the patient is mediated through the analyst's own experience." Thus, in treatments of this nature, the danger is not that analysts will lose themselves in patients' subjectivities; rather, the danger is that if analysts lack experiences that resemble those of their patients, including histories of displacement, discrimination, and violence, they will be unable to fully inhabit them.

Because so many psychoanalysts continue to contest the mutual constitution of internal and external worlds, and to deny that subjectivities are irreducibly cultural (Silver, 2017), questions such as those that are raised in my work with Z will remain unaddressed. Our work together illustrates that interior worlds of fantasy and feeling, as well as the experience of a cohesive self, take shape and continue to develop in dialogue with family histories, and with actual social and political occurrences – even though their impacts may rest outside awareness (Frie, 2012). Thus, it is crucial for psychoanalysis to recognize that the boundaries it erects to separate the individual psychic interior from political, social, and cultural conditions are mere disciplinary fabrications.

Given the inseparability of culture and mind, what violence is done to patients who are asked to collude in the fiction that when they enter the clinical space, they can leave their social and political worlds behind them? Instead of fostering integration, psychoanalysis fragments its subjects. Patients learn to silence critical areas of their personal and family histories that analysts deem irrelevant. Moreover, exclusive attention to the intrapsychic inflicts a similar violence on analysts. They too must partition their subjectivities, pushing significant aspects of their lived experience outside the clinical frame. As a result, in clinical consulting rooms, both analysts and patients are reduced to part subjects. The sway of psychoanalysis requires that both turn inward, away from the worlds that have formed them.

Then again, perhaps this is the point. As Bettelheim (1990) observed, psychoanalysis took root in the context of political and economic disaster, when a terrified populace withdrew from an environment that had turned unstable and ominous. Accordingly, despite the analytic claim that patients who discuss experiences in the external world in treatment are resisting examination of the terrors of the internal world, perhaps the opposite is true. Perhaps psychoanalysis functions as an escape from outer worlds that are intolerably treacherous and persecuting. If so, psychoanalytic inquiry is itself a resistance; a means of protecting our fragile psyches by refusing to examine exterior conditions that we cannot master or bear. When the environment feels uncontrollable, psychoanalysis offers sanctuary. It extends the comforting fantasy that irrationality and violence are safely contained inside an interior realm which analytic theory renders knowable and predictable – and in which analytic interventions produce remedial effects. We therefore should expect that in moments of catastrophe, when environments assault us, psychoanalysts will intensify their inward focus, averting their eyes from the external circumstances that sorely require their gaze.

References

Abraham, N. (1987/1994). Notes on the phantom: A complement to Freud's metapsychology. In N. Abraham & M. Torok (Eds.). *The Shell and the Kernel*, 171–176. Chicago: University of Chicago Press.

American Psychiatric Association. (1980). *Diagnostic and Statistical Manual of Mental Disorders*, 3rd Ed. Washington, DC: American Psychiatric Association.

Aron, L. & Starr, K. (2013). *A Psychotherapy for the People: Toward a Progressive Psychoanalysis*. New York: Routledge.

Behrouzan, O. (2016). *Prozak Diaries: Psychiatry and Generational Memory in Iran*. Stanford, CA: Stanford University Press.

Beltsiou, J. (2016). Seeking home in the foreign: Otherness and immigration. In J. Beltsiou (Ed.). *Immigration in Psychoanalysis*, 89–108. New York: Routledge.

Bergmann, M. (1982). Recurrent problems in the treatment of survivors and their children. In M. Bergmann & M. Jucovy (Eds.). *Generations of the Holocaust*, 247–266. New York: Basic Books.

Bettelheim, B. (1990). *Freud's Vienna*. New York: Vintage.

Boulanger, G. (2002). The cost of survival: Psychoanalysis and adult onset trauma. *Contemporary Psychoanalysis 38*, 17–44.

Brennan, T. (2004). *The Transmission of Affect*. Ithaca: Cornell University Press.

Cvetkovich, A. (2012). *Depression: A Public Feeling*. Durham, NC: Duke University Press.

Danieli, Y. (1984). Psychotherapists' participation in the conspiracy of silence about the Holocaust. *Psychoanalytic Psychology 1(1)*, 23–42.

Epstein, H. (1979). *Children of the Holocaust: Conversations with Sons and Daughters of Survivors*. New York: Penguin Books.

Estroff, S. (1993). Identity, disability and schizophrenia: The problem of chronicity. In S. Lindenbaum & M. Lock (Eds.). *Knowledge, Power & Practice: The Anthropology of Medicine and Everyday Life*, 247–286. Berkeley: University of California Press.

Fassin, D. & Rechtman, R. (2009). *Empire of Trauma: An Inquiry into the Condition of Victimhood*. Princeton, NJ: Princeton University Press.

Figley, C. R. (Ed.). (1995). *Compassion Fatigue: Coping with Secondary Traumatic Stress Disorder in Those Who Treat the Traumatized*. New York: Brunner/Mazel.

Fresco, N. (1984). Remembering the unknown. *International Review of Psycho-Analysis 11*, 417–427.

Freud, S. (1896). The aetiology of hysteria. In *The Standard Edition of the Complete Psychological Works of Sigmund Freud, Vol. 3 (1893–1899): Early Psycho-Analytic Publications*, 191–221. London: Hogarth Press, 1962.

Frie, R. (2012). On culture, history, and memory: Encountering the "narrative unconscious". *Contemporary Psychoanalysis 48*, 329–343.

Gilman, S. (1993). *Freud, Race and Gender*. Princeton, NJ: Princeton University Press.

Hartmann, H. (1958). *Ego Psychology and the Problem of Adaptation*. New York: International Universities Press.

Hoffman, E. (1999). The new nomads. In A. Aciman (Ed.). *Letters of Transit*, 39–63. New York: The New Press.

Hutchison, E. & Bleiker, R. (2008). Emotional reconciliation: Reconstituting identity and community after trauma. *European Journal of Social Theory 11*, 385–403.

Jacoby, R. (1983). *The Repression of Psychoanalysis: Otto Fenichel and the Political Freudians*. Chicago: University of Chicago Press.

Kakar, S. (1985). Psychoanalysis and nonwestern cultures. *International Review of Psycho-Analysis 12*, 441–448.

Kardiner, A. (1941). *The Traumatic Neuroses of War*. Washington, DC: National Research Council.
Kohut, H. & Wolf, E. (1978). The disorders of self and their treatment: An outline. *The International Journal of Psycho-Analysis 59*, 413–425.
Krystal, H. (Ed.). (1969). *Massive Psychic Trauma*. New York: International Universities Press.
Kuriloff, E. (2001). A two-culture psychology: The role of national and ethnic origin in the therapeutic dyad. *Contemporary Psychoanalysis 37*, 673–681.
Kuriloff, E. (2014). *Contemporary Psychoanalysis and the Legacy of the Third Reich: History, Memory, Tradition*. New York: Routledge.
Lacan, J. (1996). *Écrits*. New York: W.W. Norton and Company.
Mahler, M. (1967). On human symbiosis and the vicissitudes of individuation. *Journal of the American Psychoanalytic Association 15*, 740–763.
Mahler, M. & Stepansky, P. (1988). *The Memoirs of Margaret S. Mahler*. New York: Free Press.
Makari, G. (2008). *Revolution in Mind: The Creation of Psychoanalysis*. New York: Harper Collins.
Masson, J. (1984). *The Assault on Truth: Freud's Suppression of the Seduction Theory*. New York: Harper, Strauss & Giroux.
Mitchell, S. (1993). *Hope and Dread in Psychoanalysis*. New York: Basic Books.
Morin, E. (2001). *Seven Complex Lessons in Education for the Future*. Paris: UNESCO.
Niederland, W. (1968). The problem of the survivor. In H. Krystal (Ed.). *Massive Psychic Trauma*, 8–22. New York: International Universities Press.
Prince, R. (2009). Psychoanalysis traumatized: The legacy of the Holocaust. *American Journal of Psychoanalysis 69(3)*, 179–194.
Public Affairs Alliance of Iranian Americans (PAAIA). (2014). *Iranian Americans: Immigration and Assimilation*. http://paaia.org/wcontent/uploads/2017/04/iranian-americans-immigration-and-assimilation. Accessed 20.04.2017.
Quinn, S. (1984). Psychoanalysis and the Holocaust: A roundtable. In S. Luel & P. Marcus (Eds.). *Psychoanalytic Reflections on the Holocaust: Selected Essays*, 209–229. New York: Ktav.
Seeley, K. (2008). *Therapy after Terror: 9/11, Psychotherapists, and Mental Health*. New York: Cambridge University Press.
Shephard, B. (2000). *A War of Nerves: Soldiers and Psychiatrists in the Twentieth Century*. Cambridge, MA: Harvard University Press.
Shorter, E. (2015). The history of nosology and the rise of the *Diagnostic and Statistical Manual of Mental Disorders*. *Dialogues in Clinical Neuroscience 17(1)*, 59–67.
Shweder, R. (1991). *Thinking through Cultures: Expeditions in Cultural Psychology*. Cambridge, MA: Harvard University Press.
Silver, C. (2017). Erich Fromm and the making and unmaking of the socio-cultural. *Psychoanalytic Review 104(4)*, 389–414.
Strozier, C. (2001). *Heinz Kohut: The Making of a Psychoanalyst*. New York: Other Press.
Thompson, C. (1950/1984). *Psychoanalysis: Evolution and Development*. New York: Da Capo Press.
Thompson, N. (2012). The transformation of psychoanalysis in America: Émigré analysts and the New York Psychoanalytic Society and Institute, 1935–1961. *Journal of the American Psychoanalytic Association 60(1)*, 9–44.
Young, A. (1995). *The Harmony of Illusions: Inventing Post-Traumatic Stress Disorder*. Princeton, NJ: Princeton University Press.

6

WESTERN CONFIGURATIONS

Ways of being

Salma Siddique

Introduction

During my time as an undergraduate in the mid-1990s, I was in the fortunate position of finding myself studying under the watchful eyes of Joanna Overing (American), Ladislav Holy (Czechoslovakian) and Sandor Hervey (Hungarian-born linguist) who all congregated at the University of St Andrews, Scotland. Many times over the years we were brought together over Lévi-Strauss (1968) seminal essays "The effectiveness of symbols" and "The Sorcerer and his Magic" (1963). I had only been able to access and read from the English edition of *Structural Anthropology*: a core text for the Social Anthropology degree. It wasn't until my doctoral research into mental health and psychopathology that I really appreciated my own lived experience and what Levi-Strauss called the 'shamanistic complex' as "the faith and expectations of the group, which constantly acts as a sort of gravitational field within which the relationship between sorcerer and bewitched are located and defined" (1963, p. 168). Lakoff (2002) refer to "the structured communication between doctor and patient activates a therapeutic potentiality that exists within individuals". In the therapeutic setting, it is said that "the drug can be both a substance and symbol, and this duality is one of a number of elements that cannot be neatly tangled" (2002, p. 73). In Holy's lecture, he evoked Levi-Strauss's curing ritual performed among the Kuna Indians of Panama during a moment of a difficult childbirth (he elaborates this point even further): "what she does not accept are the incoherent and arbitrary pains which are an alien element in her system but which the shaman, calling upon myth, will integrate within a whole where everything is meaningful" (1963, p. 198). I was entranced by the power of the words and the creative images and symbols of meaning within other cultural groups. I was keen to know more. I wanted to explore these symbols and meanings as well as the spaces between things for the similarity between these two texts. I was impressed by the potentiality of the inner world meeting the outer world through the lens of anthropology.

W.H. Rivers (1864–1922) was the founding father of ethnology and ethnography: a methodology which embedded moments of lived experience understood as trauma. This theme was carried forward by Malinowski(1913) and Radcliffe-Brown (1912). However, it was Levi-Strauss (1963) who really conceptualised these moments of intrasubjective disturbance and rupture as performative and symbolic efficacy (Siddique, 2012). Rivers (1911), in the profession of psychiatry and at a time of the dawning of psychoanalysis, understood about working with his own vulnerability, as we, as therapists and at times as anthropologists, now realise the importance of the sharing of ourselves. Anthropologist and ethnopsychoanalyst Devereux (1967) suggests that "the subjectivity inherent in all observation [is] the royal road to an authentic, rather than fictitious, objectivity . . . defined in terms of what is really possible, rather in terms of 'what should be?' " (196: xviii). So, whoever the observer is, they are bringing themselves into their perspective of the helping process. My childhood was partially in Birmingham, then as a teenager in Scotland. As a first-generation Muslim, I was filled with stories of angels (malayka) made of light while the hidden spirits (jinns) were shaped from fire. I loved listening to the fascinating tales of benevolent spirits who were also prone to trickery. Often, these jinns lured disbelievers to their deaths, much like the fragmented myth of the sirens (Blanchot and Josipovici, 1982). For me, these jinns represent the 'absent presence' across the two domains of anthropology and psychotherapy and give me an understanding of people's different ways of meaning making. This was my cultural upbringing. Is it any different from transference and countertransference in psychotherapy and Freud presenting the past to work through things in the present on an individual and collective level? In my psychotherapeutic work, I am beginning to see the space between anthropology and psychotherapy. In the case of anthropology, we use objects to think with, and in the case of psychoanalysis and psychotherapy, we use objects to work through.

During my own training as a psychotherapist, I was filled with moments of anxiety and ambivalence. Mckenzie-Mavinga (2003) observed that "black issues are rarely addressed in a normative routine way"; the feelings of being missed were never engaged in dialogue within the group process or the skills work in triads. A sense of oppression and resistance remains to this day. On one occasion I arrived late, only to be met with a discussion about early childhood attachment and care from a significant caregiver. This led to a spirited and emotional exchange about anecdotal stories of poor mothering and neglect. When I wasn't able to engage with such stories, there was little attention and space given to my cultural expression of feeling the family being shamed if I discussed my parenting in such terms. Comments such as 'in denial', 'resistance' or 'repressed memories' warranted a barrage of concern over my readiness to practice as a trainee therapist. At the start of my third year, another black student joined and while introducing ourselves in the training group, she announced she was the only black woman in the group. I felt silenced by her and the rest of the group and became aware of the lack of reflexivity (intersubjective dynamics and subjective responses) in this group and generally in training about multiculturalism, now seen as a tick box exercise rather than realising that each of us brings and makes our own culture in relationship with others (Devereaux, 1963, 1969). Over the years, these stories have become experiences of black and minority ethnic supervisees I have worked with. This experience was identified in the research by Mckenzie-Mavinga (2003,): negative counselling training experiences for black and minority ethnic psychotherapy students on post-graduate courses.

It feels as if black and minority ethnic students or clients are not seen as themselves. It reminds me of the work of Zizek (2005), recalling the story of the empty wheelbarrow. A worker is suspected of stealing on leaving the factory, with an empty wheelbarrow he was rolling in front of him. The guard on the entrance gates carefully inspects and acknowledges the wheelbarrow is empty. This interaction occurs repeatedly over a number of weeks until it is realised that what the worker was stealing were the wheelbarrows themselves. Are we looking at the thing in itself, or is it just a container? It only becomes something on recognition. It is a process I am really familiar with when working with refugees. Should we not be looking at what people carry in themselves? I aim to do that in the blending of my roles as an anthropologist and as a therapist.

My experience as a psychotherapist brings together these different perspectives on therapy, which we have gained from anthropology as well as my recognition of the subjectivity of human experience as an exploration of myth making (Devereaux, 1963; Lévi-Strauss, 1978) and of reclaiming hidden objects. I see culture now as embracing all of the perspectives from the observer and the observed. Ethnography can explore more fully the unseen and the unspoken, i.e. the space between things, the fantasy relationships in the therapy room between people and between objects and the ellipses (Siddique, 2017) Here, I am using the definition of ellipsis as used in modern social technologies, meaning hesitation, intention or suspension. I see the concept of ellipsis (Calgett, 1959, p. 197) as expressing a range of linguistic and social phenomena, where the missing material can be recovered within the therapy session. The ellipsis is "in effect a space between the body and language" (de Certeau, 1988, p. 224); the metaphor is used as a way of illuminating personal identity and the professional role between therapist and client. The creation and interpretation of the space can be a felt sense of diverse words and /or gestures and movements which offer the possibility of coexisting with the other. These ideas can be seen to what Winnicott (1974, p. 51) referred to as "a reparative potential space" and a "perverse play space for discovery". This can generate meaning through the observer and the observer's internal process, which can be helpful for self-awareness and professional development. These spaces, which open up between the intersubjective, interpersonal and internal, provide a gap in gaining greater insights. This is where the real creativity lies.

I will explore these concepts of '*ellipses*' and 'space between things' and how relevant and useful they can be for our practice as psychotherapists (Siddique, 2017). In this case, I am using the term ellipsis in its grammatical meaning of omission, hesitation or pause, usually giving an element of contextual clues, and indicated in text by a sequence of three points (. . .). Herodotus is deemed by many as the originator of ethnography and refers to ethnography as the science and the art of persuasion. His monograph entitled *Histories* is usually considered as discourses relating to foreign identities and difference. Themes of these are magnified in other ethnographical informed writings such as Ondaatje (2011), who offers a style of remembering and recognising through the anthropological gaze.

The concept of culture provides a methodological and theoretical focus of social processes through which individuals make sense of their world to give shape to identities, beliefs and values through interaction. It is in the present tense about self in relation with others and through past tense when reflections and recollections of previous memory or events have the ability to transcend place, space and time: "our past is present in us as a project" (Proshansky, Fabian and Kaminoff 1983). Nationality and identity are mapped through cultural artefacts, and motifs of emotional geographies map the connection of history between body and mind. It was the work of Turnbull (1987) which informed my own ethnographical psychoanalytical style of reflexive writing and research.

In essence, I am trying to write about the space between anthropology and psychotherapy, and if this is culture in itself. Or is it more elusive? My thinking embraces the ethnographical approach from the perspective of both life-worlds and worldviews embedded in the traditions of existentialism and phenomenology, which inform the intersubjective negotiation relationship, rooted to being-in-the-world (Heidegger, 1978). This approach of ethnography and therapy supports the revealing of the ethnographers' and therapists' "prejudices, ontological assumptions, and emotional dispositions" (Jackson, 2002). But what of 'insight'? I see this as ways of being and ways of making meaning and offering discovery. The ethnographic encounter has some similarities to the therapeutic supervisory process. The therapist work is about doing, and supervision is about being. It is about finding the ethereal voice of 'being here' while embodying the experience of 'being there' (Geertz, 1988).

Absent 'presence'

My work as an anthropologist and therapist is about imagining community and challenging essentialist views of identity through exploring intra-group difference, working through what Freud referred to as "moments of collective trauma and oppression".

Freud (2010) wrote about one of his own traumas when he witnessed an event where his father was shamed but nothing was said or acknowledged:

> At that point I was brought up against the event in my youth whose power was still being shown in all these emotions and dreams. I may have been ten or twelve years old, when my father began to take his views upon things in the world we live in. Thus it was, on one such occasion, that he told me a story to show me how much better things were now than they had been in his days "When I was a young man", he said, "I went for a walk one Saturday in the streets of your birthplace; I was well dressed, and had a new fur cap on my head. A Christian came up to me and with a single blow knocked off my cap into the mud and shouted: 'Jew! get off the pavement!" "And what did you do?" I asked. "I went into the roadway and picked up my cap", was the quiet reply. This struck me as unheroic conduct of the part of the big strong man who was holding the little boy by the hand. I contrasted this situation with another which fitted my feelings better: the scene in which Hannibal's father Hamilcar Barca, made his boy swear before the household altar to take vengeance on the Romans. Ever since that time Hannibal had had a place in my phantasies.
>
> *(pp. 218–219)*

Another example of witnessing (absent presence) but not being able to intervene or make sense of it at the time was Fanon's (1952) experience, which he writes about in *Black Skin, White Masks* (1986). He describes being called out to on the street by a French child and "sees himself being seen":

> Look a Negro! . . . Mama, see the Negro! I'm frightened. . . . I could no longer laugh, because I already know there were legends, stories, history and above all historicity. . . . Then assailed at various points, the corporal schema crumbled its place taken by a racial epidermal schema. . . . It was no longer a question of being aware of my body in the third person but in a triple person. . . . I was responsible for my ancestors.

In my own case as a young child about 5 years of age, I was accompanying my mother with my 4-year-old brother to the shops a few streets away from the family home in a culturally diverse area of Birmingham, England. My mother was dressed in a traditional Pakistani Punjabi shalwar kameez with headscarf. Two skinheads were walking parallel to us on the opposite site of the road. They suddenly took sight of us before my mother had a chance to hurry us further along the road. One skinhead crossed the road and suddenly towered over us. He pushed or slapped my mother to the ground and spat at her, calling us Pakis, before rushing back over the road, and both he and his friend began laughing; they ran to the far corner of the pavement and disappeared. When I turned to my mother, she was sitting on the ground looking quite stunned with my crying brother clinging to her neck. Out of fear for myself and concern for her I asked what happened . . . why did that man hit you . . . ? Her response as she pulled herself upright was to laugh and say, "no, he didn't hit me. . . . I just slipped . . ."

These violent events are moments that mark us all as '*other*' from society. The relational configuration of enduring feelings of shame and humiliation have a profound impact on our ways of relating. Miller and Stiver (1995) correctly identified how

> we become so fearful of engaging others because of past neglects, humiliations, and violations . . . we begin to keep important parts of our experience out of connection. We do not feel safe enough to more fully represent ourselves in relational encounters.
>
> *(1995, p. 1)*

I am reminded of my work as a therapist working with anthropologists returning from the field who are not able to write up their report or thesis. They have often witnessed events encountered in the field which triggered unresolved experiences of feeling silenced, humiliated, marginalised, rejected or demeaned, and these experiences may result in disrupting or disconnecting them from initiating, maintaining or being responsive in meeting vulnerabilities and imperfections with a degree of authenticity. Most of us have experienced some traumatic events in our childhood, perhaps not as vivid as these examples of identity and ethnicity. With this in mind, I want to show how ethnography offers an awareness of the relational dynamics of these experiences. The therapy process, much like ethnography, can offer the absent presence the opportunity for negotiation of difference from "irreconcilable affections, identifications, and places of personal anchorage" (Jackson, 2012, 2002).

My experience of anthropology, which I bring to my present role as Director of Counselling and Psychotherapy Training and Research, has enabled me to embed the reflexive approach across all the programmes. Students and tutors are encouraged to reflect on their personal experiences and meanings of their understanding of culture through conceptualising bricolage (Lévi-Strauss, 1962) and to recognise and appreciate the diverse and complex negotiations which influence meaning making. I like to focus especially on how recognition and memory operate in the context of contemporary issues of belonging through dialogical processes that are socially, culturally, morally and historically embedded, and how the work of therapy (re)imagine, (re)negotiates, (re)generates and re-configures (Warner, 1991) kin and other intimate relationships to survive during contemporary times of migration, displacement and marginalisation.

Auto-ethnography in clinical practice

Auto-ethnography is about creating a self-story wherein one can maintain one's vulnerability as well as one's power; the act of writing such a story can in itself be transformative, creating "spaces for thinking about the social that elude us now" (Richardson, 2000, p. 930). Auto-ethnography therefore offers us the chance to adopt a relational perspective, so as to understand the individual in relation to their context and to look at what space is created between the therapist and client. This could be emotional, psychological, social–cultural or engendered space. At the heart of the relational research methodology is an honest, compassionate conversation about ourselves and our failings, a space where "we take measure of our uncertainties, our mixed emotions . . . and the difficulties of coping and feeling resolved, showing how we changed over time as we struggled to make sense of our experience" (Ellis and Bochner, 2000, p. 748).

The process of creating the text can give us an opportunity to present the whole of ourselves. Tierny (1998) suggests that "auto-ethnography confronts dominant forms of representation and power in an attempt to reclaim, through self-reflective response, representational spaces that have marginalised those of us at the borders" (p. 18). It is a blurring of methodology between the researcher and the researched. It encourages questioning from a wider social context and seeks to make meaning out of culture, events and life experience.

Auto-ethnography is fundamentally concerned with the therapeutic and epistemic potential of empty space. It is an intersubjective process of accounting for what happens between us, seeing the cultural scripting of participants and those who observe them as an interconnected web of relationships. These co-constructed narratives can evoke ways in which experiences are made meaningful through "effects that linger – recollections, memories, images, feelings – longer after a crucial incident is supposedly finished" (Bochner, 1984, p. 595). Auto-ethnography is an act of immersion in the very thing under investigation. In contrast to the 'evidence-based' culture of recent times, auto-ethnography does not attempt to validate rigidly structured theoretical propositions but instead responds to biographical disruptions, blind spots and fragments of social remembering through the relationship of subjective experience and space.

Ogden (1993) explores the notion of the potential space between mother and infant, which emerges through the developing awareness of where one individual ends and the other begins. According to Ogden (1993), this process of division takes place through a process of negotiation bounded by the cultural context. The infant, in this instance, is an interpreting subject who seeks to explain the behaviours and beliefs of others through projective identification. Similarly, the ethnographic collection of reflexive accounts and distant memories, which we ourselves re-author (Rabinow, 1977), re-establishes the capacity of the dialectical process to be a mode of 'thick description' (Geertz, 1973). Moutsou (2011, p. 232) has already pointed to a number of examples of anthropologists developing in dialogue with the people they studied. For ethnographers, living within the environment of study and interacting/conversing with their informants in their everyday lives can lead to transference, resistance and countertransference between anthropologist and informant (Robben, 1996), which in turn makes and unmakes spaces of displacement and/or projection. In this, it is similar to the dynamic between the analyst and analysand in terms of interpretational interventions, degrees of manipulation of relationships, developing awareness and witnessing of affect, shame, guilt and blame. As Vygotsky (1981) remarks: "It is through others that we become ourselves". Mitchell (1993, p. 132) has illuminated how the individual is co-created from relational milieus in a way that is similar to the ethnographical encounter:

> The individual discovers himself within an interpersonal field of interactions in which he has participated long before the dawn of his own self-reflective consciousness. The mind of which he becomes self-aware is constituted by a stream of impulses, fantasies, bodily sensations, which have been patterned through interaction and mutual regulation with caregivers.
> *(p. 132)*

According to psychoanalysis and psychotherapy, transference becomes 'the object of treatment', and in ethnography we explore how we understand relatedness through conceptual frameworks of 'being here' (proximity) and 'being there' (distance) that are created through the flows and counterflows that take place between ethnographer and informant; similarly, the resonance between therapist and client in their meeting makes space for each subject's reflexivity about their intersubjectivity. The space that exists between the therapist and the patient should also be considered, taking into account cultural and social norms and standards (Bollas, 2003, 2011). As we remarked earlier, there is an act of creativity which uses the empty space to make meaning: "Thirty spokes joining together at one hub/But it is the hole in the centre that makes it operable" (Laozi, 1988; see also Crapanzano, 1994, p. 236).

I find that this way of using auto-ethnography can offer the researcher/therapist an accurate picture of the therapeutic process and the lived reality of that fluid process. Rescher (2000, p. 13) refers to experiences from which "insights emerge through collective assemblage through dialogue between informants". Lévi-Strauss (1962) refers to such orderings of experiences, events, things and processes as materials (real or imagined) which are retrieved or gathered together to make a new identity or a possible subversive meaning. Derrida remarks that "if one calls *bricolage* the necessity of borrowing one's concept from the text of a heritage which is more or less coherent or ruined, it must be said that every discourse is *bricoleur*" (1978, p. 360). The counsellor or psychotherapist, as much as the client, creates a co-constructed narrative with what is available. Hatano and Wertsch (2001) discuss the ideas of assembly and *bricolage*, proposing that the "mind develops by incorporating the community's shared artefacts accumulated over generations" (2001, p. 78), which develop unequally as a discourse of the marginalised and oppressed, opening up a 'third space'. The therapy room is the liminal space between the outside world and the life-world of the client. The third space is an in-between realm devoted to the 'discourse of dissent', a space where for fifty minutes or an hour the defined and the definer are free to be '*embodied in their particularity*' (Bhabha, 2004), and that moment is witnessed.

As an academic who spends her time teaching a range of research-methods approaches to other caring professionals, I have found that using my earlier experience of fieldwork in anthropology presents ideas for enhancing the written work which would address the 'space between things' at the same time as it respects the client's narrative. The ethnographical approach goes beyond the beyond the mere act of storytelling to create an experience of the 'field' through an analysis of field and headnotes to generate insights. An ethnographic approach gave me a clearer way of expressing myself and the participatory process I underwent in observing the self in its relations with the 'other'. It helps to address the space between things and the feeling of in-between-ness itself (Siddique, 2011).

The space between things

> Doors and windows are cut
> To make a room
> It is the empty spaces that we use
> Therefore, existence is what we have,
> But non-existence is what we use.
>
> Clay is moulded into a pot,
> But it is the emptiness inside
> That makes it useful
>
> – *Laozi (cited in Zhu Xiao, Johnson, 2012)*

This extract from a poem by Laozi is suggestive of the function of empty or negative space – space held in place to create a boundary, giving shape to the wall of a building or the skin of clay pot. The disciplines of anthropology and psychotherapy speak of the potential inherent in empty space, and authors have described the way in which ritual interactions allow for emptiness. Empty space has been seen as fundamental to *basins of attraction* (Deacon, 2006), and as an essential quality of a society that tends to self-organise, or, conversely, that is in a state of collective fragmentation.

The space between things, like the 'hole in the wheel' of dynamic self-sustaining systems (Deacon, 2006), can act as a principle of attraction and organisation and so give rise to meaning and order. There is much to be learned in this respect from ways of relating which are natural, mutual and self-organising, and which are sensitive to the complexity of the modes of interaction between the subjective self and external objects. I suggest that we hold onto the essence of qualitative inquiry and so retain our sense of the fragility of these relationships, rather than adopt the universalist and explicit language of big-data-driven humanities, which tends to obscure or pass over this fragility.

As an anthropologist and psychotherapist, I consider fieldwork in and out of the therapy room as a process and as an interaction. I see the emerging material as framed autobiographical narratives of the self. Geertz (1973) remarked, following Max Weber, that

> man is an animal suspended in webs of significance he himself has spun. I take culture to be those webs, and the analysis of it to be therefore not an experimental science in search of law but an interpretative one in search of meaning. *(p. 5)*

As psychotherapists, what we observe is a web of relationships which is woven through rituals, interactions and transactions. For me, collecting stories in the field of psychotherapy and counselling is a process of writing and creating the text of the individual's lived experience – what passes between the researcher/therapist and the client is a hermeneutic-dialectic method of inquiry (Gadamer, 1999) which explores human behaviour and belief understood as a socially constructed truth. In order to understand a human being, one should aim for, to use Gadamer's expression, 'a fusion of horizons' – combining different aspects that shape our understanding of the world we live in and our behaviour in it.

The everyday world in which we live as individuals, and in which we work as psychotherapists, is evoked into 'reflective consciousness' through engaging in the act of interpretation. The act of interpretation makes and unmakes things, explicitly conceiving of the object as being in the foreground or blurring it into the background through our experience of and relationship to the object in terms of its purpose or usefulness. These practices and relationships make for 'intersubjective encounters', which Heidegger (1978) refers to as *Dasein* ('being there', 'presence' or 'existence'), the space in which meaning and truth is arrived at through forging consensus "between judgement and the world" to arrive at understanding.

Ethnographical examples from fieldwork in anthropology and psychotherapy

An example of combining of auto-ethnography with insights of 'others' is the work of French author, surrealist and ethnologist Michel Leiris (1934), who already in the early 1930s realised the value of combining his personal ('being there') and professional presence, first during the Dakar-Djibouti expedition, and later in his more detailed accounts on the Gondar of Ethiopia, as well as French Antilles (Leiris, Jamin and Mercier, 1996; Bošković, 2003). The paradox of the encounter between different worlds as different cultures is nicely summed up in a quote from his diary.

> Right away this afternoon I go with Abba Jérome to see [the Ethiopian woman] Emawayish and give her pens, ink, and a notebook so she can record for herself – or dictate to her son – the manuscript [of her songs], letting it to be understood that the head of the expedition, if he is pleased, will present her with the desired gift.
>
> Emawayish's words this afternoon when I told her, speaking of her manuscript, that it would be especially good for her to write down some love songs like those of the other night: *Does poetry exist in France?* And then: *Does love exist in France?*
>
> *(Cited in Clifford, 1988, p. 129)*

By embedding the auto-ethnographical approach into the clinical encounter, this method "allows the reader (and the writer) to experience something new – to feel, to learn, to discover, to co-create" (Ricci, 2003, p. 594).

I have worked with refugees and asylum seekers who come to psychotherapy to get a report to authenticate their experiences and to support their application to stay in the UK

As a practitioner, I have chosen a phenomenological inquiry approach to explore the relational self and identity in order to access an understanding of another's psychological health through social interaction, social reproduction and self-awareness. I choose to create a mini ethnography, which is a means to conserve an old identity while allowing for the creation of a new identity through a range of subjective, intersubjective, constructed and inherent configurations depending upon the context and the relative privilege each of these interactions allow for. At times in the process of therapy, there is a readiness to abandon, exploit or destroy the individuals' self-concept, efficacy, access to well-being and associated cultural resources.

An illustration from my own practice is a vignette I have called *Sweet and Sour*

> Qasim was a 25-year-old male Muslim refugee who was referred by his GP for low mood and withdrawal from engaging with his social space and the public environment. He claimed instantly on meeting me and my confirming that I was to work with him that we could communicate through the 'street' dialect of Sikh Punjabi, an Indo-European tonal language from an area across the Punjab and Chandigarh region.
>
> We used creative elements such as drawing, noting down observations from both the therapist and the client and then reflecting upon the writing done before, between and during the sessions to offer self-reflection and insight to cultural practices of being a young gay Muslim man in Lahore.
>
> Qasim worked on his emotional blockages through identifying different 'configurations of self' or modes of being. He often spoke about how being a gay man in an Islamic country such as Pakistan was configured differently. Qasim realized he was gay after an encounter with a boy at the local high school in Lahore, Pakistan. In this area homosexuality was based on perceptions of behaviour, religious obligations, class and family obligations in a patriarchal society. "I found it easy to be a silent author narrating my existence as though a mime, to exist between the silences and invisibility and hope not to be discovered too soon", spoke Qasim as he rested a finger on a black and white photocopy of a photograph of a scene from a Mela in which a group of men stood under a cedar tree laughing. As the conversation developed during the course of the therapy, Qasim produced more bits of paper and photographs from a carrier bag and what began to emerge was that this was his opportunity to curate the fragmentations of his past life by illuminating the differences from the insider to a changing perspective of being between cultures. He was attempting to trace his everyday lived experience in the recent past. In the following session a week later Qasim continued to express a sense of awe into his own

cultural insights about 'living creatively, living two lives . . . [he shakes head and he breaks with my gaze and looks out the window] and the other life is lived with dishonesty most of all to ourselves'. I felt he was marking the absence of presence. By crossing gender, sex and sexuality, this could be seen as a way of organising his experience as a constructed identity. Definitions of masculinity and femininity for sweet and sour, in the Sikh Punjabi language, are *Miṭhē*, which denotes sweet, while *Khaṭā'ī* refers to sour. The bittersweet tale following the masculine and sour path would be the 'rastaa', while the feminine/sweet would be 'raa' – the tone is softened according to the distance traced across the engendered experience. The rastaa is that of the smartphone and the raa is the apps to meet other gay men in the area. At other times Qasim referred to the contradictions of how difficult it was not to be lost between identities and found it useful to trace his identity through feminine/sweet and masculine/sour by othering one's own experiences to tolerate the differences and indifferences. He often found himself in the middle ground where there was no taste.

So began Qasim's auto-ethnographical writing as an accounting of his experiences and a way of integrating his sexuality through each fragment of shimmering cloth he had retrieved when fleeing the threat of violence and persecution in Pakistan. Each fragment and each element has gone some way to create a new configuration of the self. Qasim recited the past of a life of beauty and now he spoke about living amongst something dull and ugly longing for a future to start. Qasim is still waiting for the decision of his asylum seeker's application with the UK Home Office – whether he will be allowed to remain on the basis of sexual orientation and gender identity.

It is within this context that the ethnographical approach offers us an opportunity to explore 'being there' or 'presence' by '*getting with*', through developing relationships with people in the field and sharing their experiences to inform our understanding of their (and our) culture. For the ethnographic psychotherapist, the therapeutic relationship is the central focus when working in cross-cultural spaces. One of the most famous examples from anthropology is Bateson's study of the Iatmul in 1930s (Bateson, 1958). Bateson clearly demonstrated how the spaces and relationships of the anthropologists and the peoples they study are interwoven, how they constantly change and how they are (also) a product of one's own cultural upbringing. To this day, his monograph, *Naven*, stands as one of the finest examples of critical ethnography – and it is no surprise that Bateson's work remained of interest to psychologists and psychotherapists. Bateson looked at an intergenerational authoring of experience whilst still referencing the self in relation to the other. His approach has influenced my own therapy work and writing. Reflections on the place of culture should lie at the heart of psychotherapeutic practice and process. The different ways of being and belonging comprise the space that the therapist recognises in their own and their clients' identities, and which is captured in an ethnographical moment of recognition. These are therapeutic encounters across culture, belief and ethnic spaces that are connected through cultural transference.

Relational ethics: writing culture

Of course, whatever approach to understanding the lived experience of others we adopt, it is likely to have limitations. Henrich et al. (2010) have argued that the experimental findings of a number of psychological and behavioural disciplines research have been drawn from Western, educated, industrialised, rich and democratic (WEIRD) participants, who are only "representative of 12% of the world's population", and yet the findings are routinely generalised cross-culturally. If we don't look for a broader methodological base, which considers the therapeutic relationship from different aspects, then we are in danger of doing exactly what Heinrich et al. have warned against: researching a specific group of people who have been carefully selected and generalising the findings. As a black therapist, I can see the lack of diversity and cultural differences in the therapy room, on the part of both clients and therapists. As psychotherapists and counsellors, we need to expand our awareness and understanding of our cultural differences, both as a political critique of our profession as much as a principle of sensible research. We need to work and research across disciplines and across cultures to eliminate the artificial boundaries we create in reflecting the rationalist tendencies of Western scientific thought and judgement. The social and political context of qualitative inquiry method is therefore important. The collection of data and its analysis should be considered controversial, particularly in the way we write and interpret the facts.

A new approach to our work and research might call for a degree of self-disclosure by the researcher in the public domain, which may impact on the researcher's role as therapist. If a client came across the research, how would it impact on the therapeutic relationship? Do such writings lead to feelings of insights, discomfort, identification or rejection? I came to realise that when supervisees or trainees ask to see a copy of one of my articles, I always wonder what their reaction will be and whether they will think differently about me through this kind of writing and sharing. Is it possible to write in a way that the reader can gain access to the inner life of the participants, or is there an unavoidable degree of competition about what gets interpreted and what gets left out? Ultimately, it is the ethnographer who is writing the story. Yet this visibility of the author in the eyes of the subject, a problem not shared by the authors of novels, reminds us of the potentials inherent in the space between therapist and client, and of the possibility of unexpected events emerging from that space.

Conclusion: somewhere between ellipsis and precision

On reading Paterson's poem "An Elliptical Stylus" (1993), I find it offers a phenomenological understanding and personal experience of vulnerability and hope mirroring what is explored in therapy and seeking to place it within a wider political, economic and cultural context of the ethnographical encounter. This is an extract of the poem:

> he showed me how
> he'd prime the deck for optimum performance:
> it's a lesson that I recall – how he'd refine
> the arm's weight, to leave the stylus balanced
> somewhere between ellipsis and precision,
> as I gently lower the sharp nib to the line
> and wait for it to pick up the vibration
> till it moves across the page, like a cardiograph . . .
>
> *(1993, p. 2)*

> Paterson's analogy about the stylus being the instrument to produce the voice of the individual
> reminds of the presence of space in everything. We are all on a bumpy road; the stylus jumps,
> and that is what creates the resonance. We are constantly revisiting and remembering old
> records. For the ethnographer, fieldwork offers a similar process of unfolding knowledge about
> the unconscious factors behind the encountered vunerability
>
> *(Norander, 2017)*

which therapeutic and investigative intentionally transform consciousness in the process of what Freud (2010) referred to as the 'working through'. We could see 'fieldwork as confrontation' creating the "inevitable disruption of the sense of self that both the ethnographer and even his informants may experience" (Crapanzano, 1977, p. 70). This has brought about the author reworking their thinking behind the self in relation with other. This has implications for both theory and practice for the ethnographer's interactions with the informant. My work as a therapist and anthropologist has significantly raised my awareness of what I as an anthropologist am working through with my own stuff. My ethnographical work has focused on vulnerability and marginality.

My training from a relational methodology of ethnography embeds culture in the practice of everyday interaction. Enshrined in my experience of being raised in Sufism, which understands mental well-being and mental illness as being beyond the deficit model of the western scientific paradigm of disease and disorder, I attempt to focus on the breach of communitas (Esposito, 2010; Turner,1969), which informs taboos/customs and disturbances of social configurations. Most training in Western psychological approaches do not fully embrace the clients' spiritual dimensions of life and of experience (OwusuBempah and Howitt, 1995). As a clinical anthropologist working within a therapeutic frame,

I learned from working diverse realities to offer the opportunity for a space to hold a restorative dialogue and harmonise the uncertainties experienced in the everyday (Siddique, 2012). My experience as a black academic facing regular micro-aggressions when working with diverse learners from diverse backgrounds hopefully informs my culturally relative-therapeutic work. As an academic working in the field of training potential therapists for the future, I integrate anthropology into the training as I realise the importance of the diverse ways of being in the world today.

Psychotherapy and psychoanalysis need to be understood as within the idiom of the cultural liminal space between and in the ellipsis, evocative of an absent presence of an empty fullness of being in the world, referred to by Sapir (1932, p. 236): "The true locus of culture is in the interactions of specific individuals, and on the subjective side, in the world of meanings, which each one of these individuals may unconsciously abstract for himself from his participation in these interactions". When we think of the practice and performance of therapy, we need to do so with the grammar of the ellipsis of the space between things which gives the dialogue its form. As therapists we hold on to the relationship which can give both space between and can resonate the fixity and the fluidity of the encounter.

References

Bateson, G. (1958). *Naven*. Stanford: Stanford University Press.

Blanchot, M. and Josipovici, G. (1982). *The Sirens' Song: Selected Essays of Maurice Blanchot*. IN: Indiana University Press.

Bochner, A.P. (1984). The functions of human communication in interpersonal bonding. In C.C. Arnold and J.W. Bowers (Eds.), *Handbook of Rhetorical and Communication Theory* (pp. 544–621). Boston: Allyn and Bacon.

Bhabha, H.K. (2004). *The Location of Culture*. Abingdon: Routledge.

Bollas, C. (2003). Confidentiality and professionalism in psychoanalysis. *British Journal of Psychotherapy, 20*(2), pp. 157–178.

Bollas, C. (2012). *The Christopher Bollas Reader*. London: Routledge.

Bošković, A. (2003). Michel Leiris: Ethnologist in search of meanings. *Anthropos*, (H. 2), pp. 526–529.

Calgett, M. (1959). *The Science of Mechanics in the Middle Ages*. Madison: University of Wisconsin Press.

Clifford, J. (1988). *The Predicament of Culture*. New York: Harvard University Press.

Crapanzano, V. (1977). On the writing of ethnography. *Dialectical Anthropology, 2*(1–4), p. 69.

Crapanzano, V. (1994). Rethinking psychological anthropology: A critical view. In M.M. Suarez-Orozco, G. Spindler and L. Spindler (Eds.), *The Making of Psychological Anthropology II* (pp. 223–243). Fort Worth, TX: Harcourt Brace.

Deacon, T.W. (2006). Emergence: The hole at the wheel's hub. In P. Clayton and P. Davies (Eds.), *The Re-Emergence of Emergence: The Emergentist Hypothesis from Science to Religion* (pp. 111–150). Oxford: Oxford University Press.

De Certeau, M. (1988). *The Writing of History*. New York: Columbia University Press.

Derrida, J. (1978). *Writing and Difference*, trans. A. Bass. Chicago: University of Chicago Press.
Devereux, G. (1963). Primitive psychiatric diagnosis: A general theory of the diagnostic process. In *Man's Image in Medicine and Anthropology* (Monograph 4th ed., p. 337). New York: New York Academy of Medicine.
Devereux, G. (1967). *From Anxiety to Method in the Behavioral Sciences*. The Hague: George Devereux Mouton & Co and Ecole Pratique des Hautes Etudes.
Ellis, C. and Bochner, A. (2000). Authoethnography, personal narrative, reflexivity. In N. Denzin and Y. Lincoln (Eds.), *Handbook of Qualitative Research*. Thousand Oaks, CA: Sage.
Esposito, R. (2010). *Communitas: The Origin and Destiny of Community Cultural Memory in the Present*. Stanford: Stanford University Press.
Fanon, F. (1986). *Black Skin, White Masks*, trans. C.L. Markmann [1952]. London: Pluto Press.
Freud, S. (2010). *The Interpretation of Dreams*. New York: Basic Books.
Gadamer, H.G. (1999). *Gesammelte Werke: Hermeneutik 1: Wahrheit und Methode: Grundzüge einer philosophischen Hermeneutik*. Tübingen: JCB Mohr (P. Siebeck).
Geertz, C. (1973). *The Interpretation of Cultures*. New York: Basic Books.
Geertz, C. (1988). *Works and Lives: The Anthropologist as Author*. Stanford, CA: Stanford University Press.
Hatano, G. and Wertsch, J.V. (2001). Sociocultural approaches to cognitive development: The constitutions of culture in mind. *Human Development*, *44*(2–3), pp. 77–83.
Heidegger, M. (1978). *Being and Time*. London: Blackwell Publications.
Henrich, J., Heine, S.J. and Norenzayan, A. (2010). Opinion: Most people are not WEIRD. *Nature*, *466*, p. 29. Retrieved from www2.psych.ubc.ca/~henrich/pdfs/Weird%20Nature.pdf. Accessed 20.11.2011.
Jackson, M. (2012). *Lifeworlds: Essays in Existential Anthropology*. Chicago: University of Chicago Press.
Jackson, M. (2002). *The Politics of Storytelling: Violence, Transgression, and Intersubjectivity* (Vol. 3). Copenhagen: Museum Tusculanum Press.
Lakoff, A. (2002). The mousetrap: Managing the placebo effect in antidepressant trials. *Molecular Interventions*, *2*, 72–76.
Laozi. (1988). *Tao Te Ching*. Oxford: Oxford University Press.
Leiris, M., Jamin, J. and Mercier, J., (1996). *Miroir de l'Afrique: l'Afrique fantôme, message de l'Afrique, la possession et ses aspects théâtraux chez les Ethiopiens de Gondar, précédée de la croyance aux génies Zar en Ethiopie du nord, encens pour Berhané, préambule à une histoire des arts plastiques de l'Afrique noire, Afrique noire: la création plastique: accompagnées de correspondances, textes et documents inédits*. Paris: Gallimard.
Leiris, M. (1934). *L'Afrique fantôme* (Vol. 12). Paris: Gallimard.
Lévi-Strauss, C. (1962). *The Savage Mind*. Chicago: University of Chicago.
Lévi-Strauss, C. (1963). The sorcerer and his magic. In *Structural Anthropology*. New York: Basic Books.
Lévi-Strauss, C. (1968). The effectiveness of symbols. In *Structural Anthropology 1*. Harmondsworth: Penguin.
Lévi-Strauss, C. (1978). *Myth and Meaning*. London: Routledge & Kegan Paul.
Malinowski, B. (1913). *The Family among the Australian Aborigines: A Sociological Study*. London: University of London Press.
Mckenzie-Mavinga, I. (2003). Linking social history and the therapeutic process in research and practice on black issues. *Counselling and Psychotherapy Research*, *3*(2), pp. 103–106.

Miller, J.B. and Stiver, I.P. (1995). *Relational Images and Their Meanings in Psychotherapy.* Wellesley, MA: Stone Center, Wellesley College.
Mitchell, S.A. (1993). *Hope and Dread in Psychoanalysis.* New York: Basic Books.
Moutsou, C. (2011). The fieldwork model: An anthropological perspective on the process of change in long-term psychoanalytic psychotherapy. *European Journal of Psychotherapy & Counselling, 13*(3), pp. 231–245.
Norander, S. (2017). Embodied moments: Revisiting the field and writing vulnerably. *Journal of Applied Communication Research, 45*(3), pp. 346–351.
Ogden, T.O. (1993). *The Matrix of the Mind: Object Relations and the Psychoanalytic Dialogue.* Northvale: Jason Aronson Publishers.
Ondaatje, M. (2011). *The English Patient.* London: Vintage.
OwusuBempah, J. and Howitt, D. (1995). How Eurocentric psychology damages Africa. *Psychologist, 8*(10), pp. 462–465.
Paterson, D. (1993). *Nil Nil.* London: Faber & Faber.
Proshansky, H.M., Fabian, A.K. and Kaminoff, R. (1983). Place-identity: Physical world socialization of the self. *Journal of Environmental Psychology, 3*(1), pp. 57–83.
Rabinow, P. (1977). *Reflections on Fieldwork in Morocco.* Berkeley: University of California Press, Quantum Book.
Radcliff-Brown A.R. (1912). Marriage and descent in North and Central Australia. *Man, 12*, pp. 123–124.
Rescher, N. (2000). *Process Philosophy.* Pittsburgh: University of Pittsburgh Press.
Ricci, R. (2003). Autoethnographic verse: Nicky's boy: A life in two worlds. *The Qualitative Report, 8*(4), pp. 591–597. Retrieved from www.nova.edu/ssss/QR/QR8-4/ricci.pdf. Accessed 20.11.2017.
Richardson, L. (2000). New writing practices in qualitative research. *Sociology of Sport Journal, 17*, pp. 5–20.
Rivers, W.H.R. (1911). The ethnological analysis of culture. *Science, 34*(874), pp. 385–397. Retrieved from www.jstor.org/stable/1636752. Accessed 22.11.2017.
Robben, A.C.G.M. (1996). Ethnographic seduction, transference, and resistance in dialogues about terror and violence in Argentina. *Ethos, 24*(1), pp. 71–106. Blackwell Publishing on Behalf of the American Anthropological Association. Retrieved from www.jstor.org/stable/640571. Accessed 25.08.2014.
Sapir, E. (1932). Cultural anthropology and psychiatry. *The Journal of Abnormal and Social Psychology, 27*(3), p. 229.
Siddique, S. (2011). Being in-between: The relevance of ethnography and auto-ethnography for psychotherapy research. *Counselling and Psychotherapy Research, 11*(4), pp. 310–316. Retrieved from www.tandfonline.com/toc/rcpr20/11/.VAYimVZcRuY.
Siddique, S. (2012). Storymaking: In-between anthropological enquiry and Transactional Analysis Psychotherapy. *European Journal of Psychotherapy & Counselling, 14*(3), pp. 249–259.
Siddique, S. (2017). Ellipses: Cultural reflexivity in transactional analysis supervision. *Transactional Analysis Journal, 47*(2), pp. 152–166.
Tierny, W.G. (1998). Life history's history: Subjects foretold. *Qualitative Inquiry, 4*, pp. 49–70.
Turnbull, C. (1987). *Mountain People.* New York: Simon and Schuster.
Turner, V. (1969). Liminality and communitas. *The Ritual Process: Structure and Anti-Structure, 94*, p. 130.
Vygotsky, L.S. (1981). The genesis of higher mental functions. In J.V. Wertsch (Ed.), *The Concept of Activity in Soviet Psychology* (pp. 144–188). Armonk, NY: Sharpe.
Warner, M. (1991). Introduction: Fear of a queer planet. *Social Text*, pp. 3–17.

Winnicott, D.W. (1974). Fear of breakdown. *International Review of Psychoanalysis, 1*, pp. 103–107.
Zhu, X. (2012). *The Secret Piano: From Mao's Labor Camps to Bach's Goldberg Variations*. Las Vegas: Amazon Crossing.
Zizek, S. (2005). The empty wheelbarrow. *Guardian Comment*, 19 February. Accessed 12.11.2017.

7

SPIRALING TRANSFERENCE

Ellen West and the case history

Vincent Crapanzano

> We, too, react to the patient, as do other persons in his environment. Compassion, mildness, persuasion, impatience, and anger appear one by one. Thus, it was that, in the above circumstances [living day and night for two months, as a personal physician to a patient diagnosed as suffering from schizophrenic depression], I was not only able to observe the patient but also at almost each instant I had the possibility of comparing his psychic life and mine. It was like two melodies being played simultaneously; although these two melodies are as unharmonious as possible, nevertheless a certain balance becomes established between the notes of the one and the other and permits us to penetrate a bit more deeply into the patient's psyche.
>
> Eugene Minkowski (1958)

Let me begin these fractured reflections on transference and countertransference with the following anecdote. Shortly after receiving my PhD in anthropology, I was invited to attend weekly meetings at a psychoanalytic clinic in which candidates and a group of training analysts were supposed to discuss the problems these candidates were having with their first cases. Though both the analysts and the candidates knew who I was, I was never greeted by nor introduced to any of them. They sat around a long oblong table. I sat on a couch and observed from a distance without participating in the meetings. I don't know if this arrangement had been discussed. I felt – I was made to feel – an outsider. I was immediately struck by how rarely any of them intervened as a candidate discussed his problems. It was, I thought to myself, the opposite of group therapy since there was only one "patient" and between twelve and fifteen therapists present. Were these meetings the result of what the French would call *déformation professionelle*?

The candidate at the fifth meeting I attended was a rather pudgy man in his early thirties, clearly a New Yorker, surprisingly unworldly, of moderate – or rather inhibited – intelligence, and little experience. I imagined that he had decided to become an analyst in order to be analyzed without having to admit any need for it. His patient was a 16-year-old hippie who had slept her way across the country several times. He never described her. She was abstract, bodiless, without appeal. Her sexual encounters were numbered rather than described. The analysis was getting nowhere, he confessed. His confession was a plea for help rather than for advice. The longer he talked, the more embarrassed, the more confused he became. The training analysts remained silent – cruelly, I couldn't help thinking. Finally, one of them said, "It's a problem of transference," which the candidate immediately acknowledged with some relief. The question was, whose transference? He could neither describe his patient's transference nor his own countertransference. He became wordless.

I couldn't stand the silence. The poor man was suffering. I suppose the analysts were used to such anguish. Without thinking, I blurted out, "What color was her hair?" The analysts turned in unison and looked at me for the first time, some with curiosity, some with irritation, some blankly, as in a fog. The candidate opened his mouth but still no words came out, until, pathetically, he stuttered, "I don't know." The analysts scrutinized him. "What had I done?" I would have asked myself, had I had time, but, apparently, I didn't. "Was her hair long or short?" I asked. With enormous relief, the candidate answered. "It was very long, down to her, her ass. Yes, it was brown and shiny, very shiny – and messed up, always messed up." His voice suddenly became sensual. And there followed a long highly erotic description of her, her adventures, and her sexual advances. Or were they his desired advances? He was finally interrupted by the senior analyst who said his time was up. "You know, of course, what has been holding you back?" The candidate mumbled a "yes," looked at me for the first time, and then turned away before our eyes could meet.

Can my self-surprising intervention in the candidate's account described above be understood in countertransferential terms? What fascinated me, and might well have been one of the inspirations for my interest in transference, was the spontaneity of my asking what color the patient's hair was and then whether it was long or short. I was not an active participant in the mentoring session, nor was I listening with "a third ear" to what the candidate was saying. I sympathized, indeed identified, with him, but I was in fact more interested in the analysts' passive response to him. It appeared to mirror their role in a therapeutic session. The analysts' guardedness, their extended silences, and what I took to be their self-directed empathy, seemed at times cruel. Was I in fact responding to what the candidate was describing or to the circumstance in which he (and I) found himself? Can we separate the two? What role does the language – the understanding – of transference play in their conjunction or disjunction?

I begin with this anecdote because it raises some of the themes I will cover in my reflections on transference. The first part of this chapter is theoretical. I define transference and countertransference broadly as **a redirection or transfer of repressed or unacknowledged feelings, emotions, impulses, and desires from one object (person or event), most often, but not**

necessarily, from earliest childhood, to a contemporary object – in psychotherapy to the therapist or analyst. (Compare Kernberg 1965.) I am especially interested in how the language and rhetoric used to describe and interpret transferential phenomena affects transference itself; the way they figure intent; frame the encounter and its aftermath both in terms of what it includes and excludes; define its participants; determine their exchanges; encourage expected and unexpected trains of thought and action in and out of the encounter; and promote a particular hermeneutic and, in consequence, a particular image of the human – an anthropology. I consider diagnostics and the case history as configuring responses to the transferential dynamics of the encounter and its aftermath – to the spiraling of transferential relations from analyst and patient to mentors, relatives, colleagues, strangers, and readers of the case history (Crapanzano 1992). Though the case history can be taken as closure, it can also be taken as an opening – a transfer, an exorcizing gift.

The second part relates my reflections to one of the most problematic case histories in the annals of psychoanalysis: The Case of Ellen West, written by Ludwig Binswanger, the founder of Dasein, or existential, analysis. Binswanger treated Ellen West (a pseudonym) from January 10 to March 30, 1921 before she was discharged from his family clinic in Kreutzlingen on Lake Constance in Switzerland. With her husband's assistance, she poisoned herself three days later. She was 33. Ellen had already made several attempts at suicide, which she saw as the only way to escape from her all-consuming attempt to lose weight coupled with an irresistible compulsion to eat. Binswanger diagnosed her as suffering from schizophrenia simplex. He and several of his colleagues saw no possibility of recovery. She had to be placed either in a locked ward to live out her deteriorating life or released in her husband's care with the certainty of her suicide. (As it is today, assisted suicide was not considered a crime in Switzerland.) Binswanger wrote his case study twenty years later in 1944–1945 – ostensibly to illustrate his particular approach to psychoanalysis. It is starkly impersonal. There are almost no references to Binswanger's actual exchanges with Ellen and his own reaction to her. His silence has generated a significant, at times emotionally fraught, critical literature. The implementation of Ellen's death raises moral questions that lay behind that silence and, I would argue, interpretations of transference and countertransference in at least problematic cases where therapeutic intervention is in question. However great the force of experience, prognosis – and indeed diagnosis – always leaves a residue of uncertainty.

Insofar as it is possible, my aim is to discuss transference and countertransference "from a non-transferential point of view," since Freudian psychoanalysis, like other psychoanalytic schools, has a metapsychology that is embedded within – for lack of a better term – the psychoanalytic assumption itself. As such, it justifies, if it does not replicate – with putative refinement – its target language. I am not claiming, as can be seen in my definition of transference, that metalanguages are fully independent of their target language. They can provide, however, a perspective that calls attention to presuppositions latent in subject matter that can have untoward effect. Minkowski's musical metaphors might provide a more emotionally resonant, temporally sensitive way of describing a therapeutic encounter than those cast in conventional psychodynamic terms.

There are many ways of conceptualizing "transferential phenomena" in culturally resonant ways. Consider the effect of childhood, the past, indeed of origin and replay, on the perception and interpretation of the therapeutic encounter. The priority given to early childhood experiences in Freudian analysis reflect, for example, a culturally and historically specific temporality, an archeological one, that looks for origins and, in consequence, explanations in the past – in case in point, the biographical past. The deeper one delves into the past, the surer one's (causal) explanation is. The past grounds (!) explanation through the spatialization of time in terms of depth, but this spatialization is not without cost, for it renders time static. Or perhaps more accurately, the past – history, biography – is or can be layered into periods in order to restore process and duration. (I use "layered" here rather than "punctuated" in order to emphasize the seemingly inevitable spatialization of time.) There is nothing particularly new in relating time to space or space to time. I simply want to call attention to how the former, more than the latter, figures in the interpretation of transferential phenomena.

Some psychotherapies don't lay the same weight on the past, as do classical analysts. Dasein analysts, for example, focus on their patient's and their own present situation – on their responsive "being with another," which is experienced (or metaphorized) as care and love (Boss 1983: 122–125, 237–247, 255–260; Palazzoli 1963: 162) Close readings of their case studies do, however, reveal the importance they give to the past – to childhood experiences. Conservative evangelical biblical counselors, who play a far greater role in treating the mentally disturbed than is generally recognized, argue that by focusing on their client's past, they prolong their malaise, which they see as the result of the failure to recognize Jesus's redemptive power (Crapanzano 2000: 139–146).

There are societies in which childhood, the past, origin, and replay do not have the same explanatory weight they do in Euro-American culture. When I was doing fieldwork in Morocco in the late 1960s and described the role of childhood experiences on adult life to an old Sufi, he looked at me with disbelief. How could something that had happened long ago, without any manifest connection to the present, affect the life and personality of an adult? It would be a mistake to see his response as defensive. Rather, I would relate it to a picaresque sense of personal history that is conceived of – or at least narrated as – a trajectory of singular episodes that are not necessarily connected. Emphasis is placed on contingency rather than connection, producing at times wonderment and reflecting a fatalistic but not a passive attitude toward life. If my depiction of the Moroccan's conception of a life trajectory is correct, how could the often strongly affective, at times identificatory, relationship I had with several Moroccans with whom I worked be understood in terms of our conventional life trajectory? In terms of transference? What would be the effect of our different worldviews? How would they explain, if they even thought to explain, what we would call transference? Ethnopsychoanalysts like George Devereux, Paul Parin, and Melford Spiro recognized the importance of cultural difference, but for the most part they did not depart from their psychoanalytic assumption.

I have, in fact, argued that transference understood in strict Freudian terms, as a replay of childhood experiences, cannot be applied to non-therapeutic situations. Not only are there differences in intention and expectation but there are also differences in the definition of the participants (e.g.as friends, relatives colleagues, interviewees, or casual acquaintances), in their hierarchy (as doctor and patient), in etiquette (confidentiality), and in the genre and style of discourse. Ordinary conversations are not usually self-reflective; they are subject to prevailing conventions and oral genres that focus on the purported message and not conversational rhetoric; they demand a clarity of expression and a purposefulness that discourages free association characteristic of most psychotherapy; and they do not easily accept lengthy silences followed by interpretive recastings of what has transpired. I am, of course, speaking ethnocentrically, for language etiquette varies in different speech communities, including those that share the same language.

Without denying their importance, we have still to recognize the dangers in stressing cultural differences in psychotherapy. Let me give one pertinent, if exceptionally callous, example. A psychoanalytic clinic had made an agreement with a local union to offer therapy to its members in exchange for conducting research on the use of psychoanalysis in treating what the clinicians called "working class" patients. I do not think that the analysts considered the effect of labeling their patients "working class" on their interpretation and evaluation of their treatment. I have no grounds for comparing their practice with that of their middle and upper middle-class patients, but it did seem to me, as I looked at films of their sessions – "to give [them] an anthropological perspective" – that they over-simplified their interventions, were overly cautious (several seemed fearful), and poorly disguised their sense of authority. This was confirmed as the analysts discussed the films. They referred to what they took to be impulsiveness, emotionality, and proneness to anger as characteristic of the working class. "They have a different sense of time," several remarked. "They quickly develop a positive transference that rapidly turns negative." When one of them referred to cultural difference, looking to me to confirm his observation, I pointed out that the attribution of cultural difference ought to be considered in countertransferential terms (Devereux 1953; Comas-Diaz & Jacobsen 1991). He stopped short. His colleagues' responses were divided. Several agreed with me; several were clearly irritated. Had I trespassed into their territory?

Is the role of stereotypy that different from the role of diagnostics in transference? Are those therapists who argue that diagnosis interferes with treatment, in fact, able to exclude it from their attitude toward their patients? Or, is it preferable to acknowledge the role of even an implicit diagnosis in the analysis of transference? Characterization is an inevitable, if implicit, dimension of any encounter. From my position as an outsider, I would ask whether the role of such characterizations in the interpretation of transference, as important as they may be, mask what might be even more important; namely, the punctuation of the encounter, manifestly by the analyst's interventions, as Lacan (1966: 289–322) would argue, but also by the patient's oral and silent ruminations. It is not just the patient's narrative (and the analyst's largely silent one) that determines therapeutic flow but their anticipation of response. As Lacan 1966: 289–322 and Bakhtin (1984: 181–182) have insisted, the word always demands or anticipates a response, and it is this responsiveness – as asymmetrical as it may be – that finally governs the progression of analysis. The creative – the potentially transgressive – temporality of therapy is always one of suspense – a suspense, I suggest, that is an important engine of cure, adaptation, or failure. Its counterpart is boredom or its threat.

Dialogues are always multi-dimensional. They are rarely, if ever, simply an exchange of information. Indeed, the focus on the reference masks other dimensions of the exchange. I have argued (Crapanzano 1992: 115–135) that the pragmatic function of an utterance – the way it indexes the situation in which the utterance occurs – is a primary source of the attributions and interpretations of transference. Indexical locutions – such as here, there, now, then, me, you, yesterday, or tomorrow as well as titles and tense – not only point to purportedly fixed, real, or imagined contextual features but also effect changes in our response to them, which influence the encounter and its interpretation. In a close reading of Freud's Case of Dora, I (Crapanzano 1992: 115–135) pointed out that the play between Freud and Dora's modes of address as well as how they each denominated significant figures in Dora's life influenced the development of their transference and its interpretation. Freud sometimes switched between the formal German pronoun (*Sie*) and the informal *du* in addressing Dora, just as he sometimes referred to Dora's father as *Ihr Vater* or *dein Vater* and at other times as *Ihr* or *dein Papá*. Dora also switched honorifics and references to her father.

Any dialogical engagement can be viewed as an arena in which the participants are unwittingly (at times wittingly) negotiating and renegotiating the terms of engagement: their respective identities, their authority, their dominance, the appropriate communicational genres, and conventions – including the choice of language, style of expression, affective tolerance, manner of address – and the appropriate mode of interpretation. I suggest that the psychoanalyst responds less to the referential message the patient is conveying and more to its pragmatic and affective features. These would include, insofar as it is possible, given the analyst's participation in the therapeutic dialogue, his or her own countertransferential reflections and affective responses. The analyst's focus on these pragmatic features, and others too, is facilitated by the patient's purported free associations, in which even the referentiality of the patient's words is less significant than their pragmatic weight, particularly as markers of the patient's state of mind.

But, what do we mean by the "patient's state of mind"? The loosening of speech etiquette, grammatical constraint, and narrative convention in the patient's free associations opens the way for other voices to be sounded. That is to say, the ruminations are double voiced, at times multivoiced, and shift with time. There are several ways in which a speaker (a patient in analysis) can give voice to another (Bakhtin 1984: 181ff; Lee 1997: 293–320). The most obvious is direct quotation. Frequent in literary works, it is rare in ordinary conversation and presumably in psychoanalytic sessions. When it does occur, it clearly distinguishes the speaker's words from those of the person quoted and is suggestive of the speaker's reportorial objectivity, but of course this is not quite the case because the speaker's choice of introductory expressions in the main clause reflects his or her attitude toward the quoted speaker. A speaker may say, for example, "Joan said [or cried, whispered, or stuttered, or said sadly, angrily, or gleefully], 'Mary is not attending John's wedding.'" The quoted words are recontextualized as a unit and serve rhetorically for the speaker (Joan). It also indexes the speaker's desired identity. As Bakhtin notes, "Two utterances, whatever they may be, as soon as they are set side by side on the same semantic plane (not as objects or as linguistic examples) will find themselves in a dialogical relation" (Todorov 1984: 74).

Indirect discourse is a second way of giving voice to another. If the speaker uses the phrases of the quoted speaker, there is little difference except in tense and pronominal usage between direct and indirect discourse, but, in fact, the speaker has greater freedom since he or she is usually taken to be paraphrasing, condensing, parodying, ironizing, or mirroring the style of the quoted speaker. The difference between the speaker and the quoted speaker is blurred and the quotation has less objective authority. The speaker's voice resonates in the referenced speech.

The third way of giving voice to another is free indirect discourse (*erlebte Rede* or *discours indirect libre*), which is mainly a literary device in Euro-American but not in all speech communities. The narrator takes on the speech of a character or the character takes on the speech of the narrator and the two instances are merged. Introductory expressions such as "he said" are absent. I suggest that free indirect discourse occurs when patients and analysts are so deeply immersed in their streams of consciousness that they lose narrative perspective. I have often observed this when the spirit-possessed emerge from their trance, the dreamers from their dream, and among some schizophrenics.

How do the addressees in free indirect discourse determine when speakers are speaking in their own voice (if they ever do) and when they are speaking in another's voice? How do we parse the merging – the merged – voices? The obvious answer is through style, including paralinguistic phenomena such as intonation, nasalization, pitch, rhythm, hesitations, facial expressions, and gestures. We suddenly hear speakers use words, phrases, and references that seem alien to what they have just been saying or we expect from them. We hear the echoing of another's voice, which is not necessarily the voice of any single individual, but as Bakhtin (1984: 184ff) would insist, the voice of another speech community – a particular class, ethnic group, race, or age.

It would seem that the psychoanalyst is – or should be – especially sensitive to these variant voices, just as the musical scholar is aware of musical references that the ordinary listener hears but does not recognize. What is important from a therapeutic point of view is not how the voices are distinguished but how they are heard, identified, reported in a case study, for example, and interpreted. A Freudian is likely to be attuned to hearing parental voices echoing forward from earliest childhood; a Jungian to archetypical figures emerging from the collective unconscious; and an existential analyst to cues to a patient's way of being-in-the-world. Analysts, caught up in their own ruminations, would not in all likelihood be aware of changes in their own voice, discourse forms, and indexical locutions, upon which their interpretive interventions are based.

Is it possible to speak of the communications that occur during a therapeutic session as a specifiable speech genre? Compared to written genres, oral ones are looser, less stable, and more difficult to define. Bakhtin (1986: 60) refers to their "boundless heterogeneity." Although they are constantly being negotiated and renegotiated, they are rarely at the center of a speaker's attention. Were they acknowledged, they would probably be given a fixity that would undermine the effect of their continual retuning.

Judging from how few discussions of genres, even literary ones, there are in psychoanalysis, it seems likely that they rarely figure in the interpretation of transference. Nor, as far as I can tell, is the case history seen as a symptom of countertransference and read as such. One characteristic of these write-ups, as in Binswanger's case studies, is how often they fail to reproduce or even evoke the dialogical nature of therapy. (Freud's cases, especially Dora and Rat Man, are, within the limits of his authorial control, exceptional.) As we shall see in our discussion of the Case of Ellen West, Binswanger and the two psychoanalysts who treated her rarely quote or even refer directly to their exchanges with her. The mode of reportage, including voicing or its absence, has to be understood in countertransferential terms that affect their readers' response. They produce an empty surround that facilitates imaginative constructs as well as evaluations that perhaps arise from the anxiety of not knowing. They can lead at times to egregious, moralistic, and historically insensitive misreadings. Ironically, it is Ellen in her letters and her husband Mark in his diaries who give a sense of her dialogical engagement in her several therapies.

****

> I am a prisoner in myself.
>
> *Ellen West*

Although Ellen West suffered from eating compulsions for more than ten years before she was admitted to Bellevue, she only received psychiatric help in the last year and a half of her life. She had sought help from various medical doctors but without avail. It was, however, her internist who finally insisted that she be sent to Binswanger's clinic. Bellevue had an elite clientele that, as was customary at the time, often came with family members. It is in many respects reminiscent of the Berghof in Thomas Mann's *The Magic Mountain*. Binswanger's grandfather, who had founded it in 1857, believed that the doctors' families should participate, whenever they could, in their patients' treatment by socializing with them. At 29, Binswanger became director of Bellevue after his father's death in 1910. He had previously been an assistant at the Berghölzli Psychiatric Clinic in Zurich, which was then under Jung's direction. It was Jung who introduced him to Freud, and he soon began practicing psychoanalysis and promoted it, not without controversy, as one of Bellevue's treatments. Binswanger and Freud became friends and, though they parted ways intellectually when Binswanger turned to Husserl's phenomenology and Heidegger's existentialism in the hope of grounding psychoanalysis anthropologically, they remained friends and corresponded until Freud's death. To my knowledge, Binswanger never discussed Ellen with Freud.

The publication in 1958 of *Existence*, a collection of essays on existential psychoanalysis, including the Case of Ellen West (May, Angel, & Ellenberger 1958), produced a flurry of interest among American psychoanalysts and psychotherapists, but it soon diminished because most therapists were unfamiliar with its philosophical basis and were uncomfortable with its focus on a patient's particular style of being in the world and how that style impeded the actualization of his or her authentic being rather than on therapeutic practice (May, Angel, & Ellenberger 1958: 7–10). The Italian psychiatrist Mara Selvini Palazzoli (1963: 158) puts the difference succinctly: "Existential analysis was essentially born as a psychopathology and not as a psychotherapy." She quickly adds that the recognition of the patient's mode of self-realization is the meeting point of a psychopathology of the interior (*dal di dentro*) and psychotherapy, which it enriches.

Existential psychoanalysis can be seen as a critique of positivism, its insistent pragmatism, and its rejection of the spiritual and the transcendent. It was explicitly a reaction to Freud's biologism, his postulation of an unconscious, and his mechanistic theory of the psyche. Existential analysts do, however, use many of Freud's techniques – free association, the analysis of transference, and the punctuation of the patient's discourse by interpretive interventions. The focus of their interpretations is usually on the patient's immediate situation and future aspirations.

"The Case of Ellen West" (Binswanger 1958, 1957) is at once a case history, an example of Dasein analysis, though not of its therapeutic technique, a comparison of classical psychoanalysis and clinical psychiatry, and a discussion of various approaches to schizophrenia. It can also be read as a rationalization of Binswanger's diagnosis and treatment of Ellen (Akavia 2008: 136–137). It is based primarily on Ellen's poems, which she began to write at 15, intermittent diary entries, reports from her psychoanalysts, and on an anamnesis that her husband prepared at Binswanger's request (Akavia 2008: 134–135). Binswanger does not read the poems and diary entries in terms of Ellen's age or their context. Indeed, he is quite dismissive of her literary talent (Studer 2007: 150, 164). He is exceptionally careful to guard her identity and, as I have noted, included few of his own observations of her. During the three months that Ellen was in the clinic, his contact with her was limited to two short daily visits. He prescribed rest, baths, and walks – above all patience – and told her that psychoanalysis in cases of melancholia (his first diagnosis) was useless, even harmful. In a letter to her parents, Ellen writes that despite their brevity,

> his visits and constant care are beneficial; he always lets me describe the exact course of the day and night, tries to encourage me, presses me to pour out my heart to him; gives this or that medicine to help get over the particular depressive hours.
>
> *(Akavia 2008: 124)*

Mark was usually present and mediated their encounter. (The two psychoanalysts who had treated Ellen earlier objected to his presence.) Binswanger and Mark became friends, playing music together during Ellen's stay at Bellevue. They corresponded periodically until 1961. Ellen's death was often mentioned.

Ellen's family were wealthy Jews, presumably from Germany or the Austro-Hungarian Empire. Ellen venerated her father. She describes him as self-controlled, willful, and stiffly formal – a man of action – but sensitive and soft (*weich*) inside. He was adamantly secular. Her mother was very soft, kindly, suggestible, and nervous. Binswanger (or Ellen) barely mentions her. Nor does he describe his meeting her parents. Ellen grew up in a surround of mental illness: her parents were depressive; a paternal aunt became mentally ill on her wedding day; one of her brothers had been suicidal, two of her five paternal uncles had committed suicide, two suffered dementia, and the fifth led an exceptionally ascetic life. Her paternal grandmother was manic-depressive. Interested primarily in Ellen's present life, Binswanger ignores the possible effect of this environment on her.

As a child Ellen was, by her own admission, lively, headstrong, and violent, suffering at times from a sense of unexplainable emptiness. When she was 10, her family moved back to Europe. Ellen was a good, ambitious student but remained willful, choosing as her personal motto *aut Caesar aut nihil*. At 16 she stopped sucking her thumb and began playing boys' games and even expressed the desire to be a boy in one of the many poems she started writing at the time. She sees herself as destined to achieve something special. Distraught by her privilege, she wants to help the poor. After reading Jens Peter Jacobsen's novel *Niles Lyhne*, whose esthetic individualism and religious nihilism had enormous influence among the bourgeois youth of the time, Ellen, like its hero, loses the religious faith that she had held, to Binswanger's mind, in opposition to her father and gains a stronger sense of her own individuality. (On rereading the novel, I suddenly realized the extent to which it influenced Binswanger's portrait of Ellen.)

Despite hints of darkness, Ellen seems to be happy, exuberantly so. Her poems are romantically melancholic. The desire to escape confinement – a tomb in many of her poems – and to fly freely through the air before returning to the world of small things is a leitmotif in many of her poems and becomes an organizing trope for Binswanger, who stresses her struggle between her growing sense of terrestrial – corporeal – entombment and her ethereal – unrealizable – aspirations. The one is dark, moldy, worm-ridden – the world of the grave, the bourgeois Jewish body, imaged at times as hole. The other is airy, unstable, embodying the blond, intellectual Aryan, glowing, scary in its possibility – the irreal world of flight (Bray 2001). Despite the importance Binswanger gives to the *Mitwelt* (roughly the social world) in his writings, he pays scant attention to the sociohistorical circumstances of Ellen's life. He does not relate this struggle to the constricted life of women at the time, the prevailing anti-Semitism, and the power given a father (Burstow 1980–1981).

At 18, Ellen travels to Paris with her parents and, as Binswanger (240; 64) puts it, "new little sentimental love affairs develop." It is worth noting at this point that references to the case of Ellen West from this point on will be indicated by page numbers only; the first to the English translation, the second to the 1957 German edition. At 19, she travels overseas to visit family and friends. She (241; 64–65) remembers it "as the happiest and most harmless (*harmlosest*) time" in her life, but complains that she can't escape her parents. When she returns to Europe, she takes up riding and rides dangerously. She longs for thrills, imaging in her poems "gales roaring through the world," "her blood races and roars through her veins." She imagines a lover, "tall and strong, pure of soul, who does not play or dream life, but lives it. He must enjoy her and her children" (241; 65). She becomes engaged to a riding master. Her father breaks up the affair.

Later in same the year, Ellen crosses the Atlantic again to nurse her sick brother. She becomes engaged to "a romantic foreigner" but again breaks the engagement at her father's command, apparently without much anguish. This is the last time, Binswanger notes ominously, that she enjoys eating and drinking (241; 65). On her way home, she stops in Sicily, begins to doubt herself, eats ravenously, and soon becomes so fat that her friends taunt her. Still in Sicily, she mortifies herself with fasting and excessive exercise. Thus begins a struggle that will take full possession of her. Her self-mortification will reach unheard of proportions: at one point taking thirty-eight to forty-eight thyroid pills a day and at another sixty to seventy laxatives. Her weight will vary between 90 and over 160 pounds. Periods of ever longer and more severe depressions alternate, often without manifest cause, with remissions. Death increasingly becomes her only salvation. In one of her diary entries she figures it not as a man with a scythe but as "a glorious woman, white asters in her dark hair, large eyes dream-deep and gray" (242; 66).

Ellen is not, however, without inner resources. She is acutely aware of her inner life, and even in the last days before her suicide, she remains particularly articulate about what she is experiencing. She starts children's reading rooms, engages in social work, believes in the need for revolution, studies for university entrance exams . . . but she gives them up while extolling the importance of work – her sole relief from her fixation on her weight. Again, she becomes engaged to a student with whom she seems genuinely in love. Her father discourages her until finally she marries her cousin Mark, a lawyer, who devotes himself assiduously to her, indeed leaving her little space of her own. She longs ambivalently for a child, has a miscarriage, and remains barren.

When she is 32, Ellen begins her first psychoanalysis with Viktor Emil Freiherr von Gebsattel, whom Binswanger characterized superciliously as "a young and sensitive analyst who is not completely committed to Freud" (249; 73). Judging from the letters Ellen wrote to her husband, she regains hope, begins to live again – "over-doing everything" – and develops deeper insight into the meaning of her obsessions, though the dread of getting fat remains. Six or seven months later her analysis ends – "for external reasons," Binswanger says. In fact, Gebsattel seems to have suffered a breakdown (Akavia & Hirschmüller 2007: 35–49; Scheible 2007: 176–178).

A few months later, Ellen begins analysis again, this time with a more experienced, though opinioned, analyst, named Hans von Hattingberg. She attempts suicide several times during her analysis, once trying to jump out of Hattingberg's window. In her diary, her relentless dread of becoming fat is mechanically punctuated by insights echoing Hattingberg's interpretations. She writes about herself with an objectifying perspective. There are moments of improvement followed by increasingly serious relapses. Emil Kraeplin, the famous nosologist, is called in and says she is suffering from melancholia. Ellen's analyst disagrees and continues her treatment despite her deteriorating condition. Her internist finally insists that she stop analysis and transfer to Bellevue. She is 33.

In his report to Binswanger, Hattingberg diagnoses Ellen as suffering from "a severe obsessive neurosis combined with manic-depressive oscillations." He is convinced she is on the way to recovery. He suggests that her depressions are "strongly and purposefully aggravated" and notes that her father did not understand her obsessive ideas but understood her depressions. She told Hattingberg that becoming fat would displease the student with whom she still seems to be in love and associates being thin and blond with "a higher intellectual type" and "being fat with a bourgeois Jewish type." Hattingberg was blond. She rejects both his suggestion that her hysterical traits were "calculated to impress her husband" and is equivocal about his suggestion that for her "eating = being fertilized = pregnancy = getting fat." She does develop an intense father–daughter transference with him. She suddenly sits on his lap and kisses him; she lays her head on his shoulder and asks him to call her "Ellen-child" (Akavia & Hirschmüller 2007: 141). Her analysis flags when it turns to her father. She does make clear, however that "her obsessional idea" means "turning away from the paternal (Jewish) type."

At Bellevue, Ellen's world narrows dramatically. She continues to obsess over her weight, is ever more attentive to her inner experiences, and is convinced that only death can offer her escape from her ceaseless struggle with her unfathomable compulsion that she now figures metaphorically as an irrepressive devil in her. Binswanger finally decides that she has either to be placed in a locked ward – as her husband has to return to work and cannot guarantee her safety – or leave the clinic (Akavia 2008: 125–130). He seeks confirmation of his prognosis from Eugen Bleuler, a leading expert on schizophrenia, and from "a foreign psychiatrist" (p 266; 91), who diagnoses Ellen as suffering from a "psychopathic constitution progressively unfolding." This "foreign psychiatrist" we learn in the archives was Alfred Erich Hoche, the co-author with the jurist Karl Binding of *The Permission to Annihilate Life Unworthy of Life*, which had been published with considerable sensation a year earlier and was to be used by the Nazis to justify euthanasia and the death camps. Both Bleuler and Hoche agree with Binswanger's prognosis, and Ellen is released the day of the consultation. The following two days are more harrowing for Ellen than all the previous weeks, so Karl writes Binswanger, but on the third day, she is transformed. In a festive mood, she eats with satisfaction, takes a walk with Karl, reads poetry, writes to a friend at Bellevue, and gives detailed instructions for her funeral and her legacy. In the evening she takes a lethal dose of poison and the next morning is dead. "She looks as she had never looked in life – calm and happy and peaceful" (267; 92).

The revelation of the identity of the "foreign psychiatrist" raises a number of questions about Binswanger's integrity – his decision to release her from the clinic, his enigmatic relations with her husband, and his conviction that no cure or even remission is possible. His reaction to Ellen's death is a philosophical romantic meditation on suicide, death, and the positivity of nothingness. Binswanger (292–298; 166–122) declares that, unlike her earlier attempts at suicide, this time her "suicide was 'premeditated,' resolved upon after mature consideration." In her resolve Ellen did not "grow beyond herself," but rather, in her decision for death, did she find herself and chose herself. "The festival of death was the festival of the birth of her existence. Where the existence can exist only by relinquishing life, there the existence is a tragic existence" [*Wo aber das Dasein nur zu existieren vermag unter Preisgabe des Lebens, da ist die Existenz eine tragische Existenz*] (298;122). As profound as his meditation is – and in many respects it is – it ends, as does any description of death, in inescapable cliché.

Of course, reality intervenes. Answering a letter from Binswanger, Hoche writes on April 16, 1921 that neither suicide nor assisting suicide is punishable (Akavia & Hirschmüller 2007: 159). "Had the husband not only laid down the poison for use but had injected it, so would it be 'voluntary homicide' with the potential result of a couple of years in prison – a noteworthy example of the incongruent borderline between the human and legal."

*****

> It is a tragic-comical paradox that Binswanger's account [of Ellen West] is, in many away, a perfect account of just what he is striving, not desperately enough, not self-reflectively enough and not self-ironically enough to eschew and leave behind.
>
> *Ronald Laing (1982: 54)*

As I have argued, diagnosis (or its absence) figures in the analysis of countertransference. From the very start of Ellen's psychiatric treatment, the question of her diagnosis was raised. Kraeplin diagnosed her as melancholic; von Gebsattel as an obsessive neurotic; Hattingberg as suffering from "severe obsessive neurosis combined with manic-depressive oscillations"; Binswanger changed his diagnosis from melancholia to schizophrenia simplex; Bleuler accepts Binswanger's diagnosis as schizophrenia; and Hoche, as we might expect, as "a psychopathic constitution progressively unfolding." It is noteworthy that the question of diagnosis also figures in most of the reactions to Binswanger's text – reactions that I view in spiraling countertransferential terms. Nassir Gaemi (2001) diagnosed her as suffering from bulimia nervosa with possibly a brief period of anorexia; Palazzoli (1963) from mental anorexia (anoressia mentale); Salvador Minuchin (1984) from anorexia; Caude Marceau (2002) from ontological insecurity and body shame (*honte de corps*); Manoel Berlincke and Cecília Magtas (200) a from a narcissistic neurosis resulting from a conflict between the ego and the high ideals of a severe superego (*severidade do superego*); Jean-Claude Maleval from hysterical insanity (*folie hystérique*): Akavia (2008: 119) an eating disorder coupled with a borderline disorder.

Indeed, the secondary literature on the Case is emotionally charged (Akavia 2008: 120–121). Its authors mourn Ellen; blame her family for not doing enough to allay her distress and prevent her suicide; and culpabilize her therapists, especially Binswanger, for the failure of their treatments, often ignoring the state of psychiatry at the time. Their anachronism is often egregious, arrogantly so. Carl Rogers (1989: 158–168) retells Ellen's life in simplistic, historically, and culturally insensitive terms and on the basis of *that* retelling imagines the person-centered therapy he would undertake to put her in touch with her own experiences. The circularity of his argument is exquisite! Unlike Rogers and to a lesser extent Binswanger, who seem oblivious to the real-life constraints on Ellen, other commentators stress the limitations on Ellen's – or women's – self-fulfillment given the customs of the times. Almost all the critics, notably the Americans, are particularly incensed by Binswanger's insistence that it was only through her death that Ellen was able to achieve authentic existence. They understand his position – not in philosophical terms, as presumably he had intended – but as a rationalization for discharging her. His case study was meant to be exemplary – scientific – and, despite his failure to name the "foreign psychiatrist," professionally, if not confessionally, upright. Yet, as Akavia and Hirschmüller point out, there are self-defensive omissions in his account. Nearly all the readers, even before the opening of the archives, are troubled by Ellen's husband's role in her treatment, his insistent presence in her life, his relations with Binswanger, including their decades-long correspondence, and, of course, his actual role in her suicide.

******

What is extraordinary about Binswanger's study is his dependency on written texts rather than on his actual experience of Ellen. Even his case notes are sketchy, especially when compared to those on the art historian Aby Warburg, who was admitted to Bellevue a few days after Ellen's death (Binswanger & Warburg 2006). True, Binswanger wrote the case history twenty years after Ellen's death, but to reduce his reliance on written texts to a scrupulous concern for evidence that is not subject to the distortions of memory seems evasive. Whatever the reason for his inordinate reliance on written texts – and there are no doubt many – the Case of Ellen West is a textualization of texts, some based on still other texts, including those that Binswanger himself requested (e.g. Karl's anamnesis, records from Ellen's psychoanalysts, etc.). Like all texts, even fictional ones, they distance their authors from the events they recount and the characters they describe and thereby facilitate objectification and with objectification detemporalization. Ellen becomes a "human individuality" (*eine menschliche Individualität*) in Binswanger's Dasein-analytic discussion of her case. We forget that in Liliane Studer's (2007: 149) words, Ellen was a woman "who tried to defend herself against conventions, who sought a meaningful life, saw her ideals fade away, and finally chose suicide."

Distance created by entextualization creates a gap between text and experience – between Ellen as experienced and Ellen as written, more accurately, Ellen as encountered and Ellen as recounted. There is nothing particularly new about this observation, if we understand it in structural terms. But I ask, what is the effect of this gap – this emptiness – in experiential terms? I suggest that it opens, on the one hand, the non-space–non-time of imagination where realism plays against illusion and phantasy as *they* play against realism; and, on the other hand, it produces the space–time of longing for engagement. Or, in Heidegger's terms, for care, or in Binswanger's, for love. Or, indeed, their opposites: indifference and dislike. It is, for our purposes, the where and the when of transference and its spiraling out to others.

We have to ask how a case study can figure in countertransference and its spiraling to its readership. Binswanger writes impersonally, with the then (and still) prevailing authoritative style of the German Swiss physician (as I can attest to personally), which should not be read simply as a defense of his decision to surrender Ellen to her fate. And yet his writing, especially his discussion of poetry, displays a countervening aesthetic sensibility that suggests an affective – a caring or loving – dimension to his relationship with her. But with the exception of some of her poems and diary entries, Binswanger rarely quotes her or anyone else's exchanges with her directly. Nor do her psychoanalysts. The reader is deprived of a sense of their dialogical engagement. The poems and diary entries are read fixedly as symptoms of her condition and as such the inevitable stasis – the deadened time of obsession.

The biographical sections of Binswanger's study, which follow Ellen's life trajectory chronologically, insistently so, without judgment, as Binswanger puts it, and explicit analysis, conjures up fatality. It is not just the fatality that arises from being cast in a particular world without rhyme or reason. According to Binswanger, every individual is possessed of a unique existential structure, or

Welt-Entwurf, that determines his or her way of constituting self and world. Given a-priori, as a structure rather than a potential, it delimits the individual's freedom, promotes conformity, and supports the fatality of being what one is and not what one would like to be. Ellen's being-in-the world is one of hopeless defiance. Binswanger's narrative also resonates with the "fatedness" of schizophrenia, as it was understood at the time and still hovers beneath our understanding today. In other words, Binswanger gives stylistic support to his decision to release Ellen to what has been fated. Realism prevails. Ellen comes to have the maturity, Binswanger avers, to accept what was fated. But the question remains: Was it fated?

Abetting the death of another, however justified it may be, inevitably leaves an insidious doubt that cannot – ought not, in my view – be reduced to feelings of guilt, as we are wont to do, for there is always the possibility of solace in guilt which doubt can never provide.

References

Akavia, N. (2008). Writing "the case of Ellen West": Clinical knowledge and historical representation. *Science in Context*, 21: 119–144.

Akavia, N. & Hirschmüller, A. (2007). *Ellen West: Gedichte, Prosatexte, Tagebücher, Krankengeschichte*. Kröning: Ansanger.

Bakhtin, M. (1984). *Problems in Dostoevsky's Poetics*. Minneapolis: University of Minnesota Press.

Bakhtin, M. (1986). Speech *Genres and Other Late Essays*. Austin: University of Texas Press.

Berlinck, M. & Magtaz, A.C. (2008). Reflexões sobre o caso de Ellen West: Estudo anthropológico, de Binswanger. *Revista Latinoamericana de Psicopatologia Fundamental*, 11(2): 232–238.

Binswanger, L. (1957). *Schizophrenie*. Pfullingen: Neske.

Binswanger, L. (1958). The case of Ellen West. In: May, R., Angel, E., & Ellenberger, H. (Eds.). (Pp. 237–264). *Existence: A New Dimension in Psychiatry and Psychology*. New York: Basic Books.

Binswanger, L. & Warburg, A. (2006). *La guérison infinie: Histoire clinique d'Aby Warburg*. Paris: Rivages.

Boss, M. (1983). *Psychoanalysis and Daseinsanalysis*. New York: Da Capo Press.

Bray, A. (2001). The silence surrounding "Ellen West": Binswanger and Foucault. *Journal of the British Society for Phenomenology*, 32(2): 125–146.

Burstow, B. (1980–1981). A critique of Binswanger's existential analysis. *Review of Existential Psychology and Psychiatry*, 16: 245–252.

Comas-Diaz, L. & Jacobsen, F. (1991). Ethnocultural transference and countertransference in the therapeutic dyad. *American Journal of Orthopsychiatry*, 61: 392–402.

Crapanzano, V. (1992). *Hermes' Dilemma and Hamlet's Desire*. Cambridge: Harvard University Press.

Crapanzano, V. (1996). Kevin: On the transfer of emotions. *American Anthropologist*, 96(4): 866–885.

Crapanzano, V. (2000). *Serving the Word: Literalism in America from the Prophet to the Bench*. New York: The New Press.

Devereux, G. (1953). Cultural factors in psychoanalytic therapy. *Journal of the American Psychoanalytic Association*, 1: 629–655.

Di Nicola, V. (2011). *Letters to a Young Therapist: Relational Practices for Coming Community*. New York: Apropos.

Gaemi, S.N. (2001). Rediscovering existential psychotherapy: The contribution of Ludwig Binswanger. *American Journal of Psychotherapy*, 55(1): 51–64.

Kernberg, O. (1965). Notes on countertransference. *Journal of the American Psychoanalytic Association*, 13: 38–56.

Kirschenbaum, H. & Henderson, V. (Eds.). (1989). *The Carl Rogers Reader*. Boston: Houghton Mifflin.

Lacan, J. (1966). *Ecrits*. Paris: Seuil.

Laing, R. (1982). *The Voice of Experience: Experience, Science and Psychiatry*. New York: Penguin Books.

Lee, B. (1997). *Talking Heads: Language, Metalanguage, and the Semiotics of Subjectivity*. Durham and London: Duke University Press.

Marceau, J.-C. (2002). La question de la corporéité dans le cas Ellen West de L. Binswanger. *L'Evolution Psychiatrique*, 67(2): 367–378.

May, R., Angel, E. & Ellenberger, H. (Eds.). (1958). *Existence: A New Dimension in Psychiatry and Psychology*. New York: Basic Books.

Minkowski, E. (1958). Findings in a case of schizophrenic depression. In: May, R., Angel, E., & Ellenberger, H. (Eds.). (Pp. 127–138). *Existence: A New Dimension in Psychiatry and Psychology*. New York: Basic Books.

Minuchin, S. (1984). The triumph of Ellen West: An ecological perspective. In: Minuchin, S. (Ed.). (Pp. 195–246). *Kaleidoscope: Images of Violence and Healing*. Cambridge: Harvard University Press.

Palazzoli, M.S. (1963). *L'anoressia mentale: Dalla terapia iindividuale alla terapia familiare*. Milan: Feltrinelli.

Rogers, C. (1989). Ellen West and Loneliness. In: Kirschenbaum, H. & Hendersen, V. (Eds.). (Pp. 57–168). *The Carl Rogers Reader*. Boston: Houghton, Mifflin.

Scheible, B. (2007). Viktor Emil von Gebsattel: der erste Analytiker von Elllen West. In: Hirschmûller, A. (Ed.). (Pp. 171–180). *Ellen West – Eine Patientin Ludwig Binswangers: Zwischen Creativität und destructivem Leiden*. Kröning: Ansanger.

Studer, L. (2007). Schriftstellerin oder Anorektikerin? Ellen West in Spannungsfeld von eigenen Wünschen und gesellschaftlichen Erwartungen. In: Hirschmûller, A. (Ed.). (Pp. 149–169). *Ellen West – Eine Patientin Ludwig Binswangers: Zwischen Creativität und destructivem Leiden*. Kröning: Ansanger.

Todorov, T. (1984). *Mikhail Bakhtin: The Dialogical Principle*. Minneapolis: University of Minnesota Press.

AFTERWORD

Sudhir Kakar

The stimulating chapters in this book took me back to my own training analysis almost fifty years ago. After some months of five-day-a-week analysis with a German analyst at the Sigmund-Freud Institut in Frankfurt, I realized that my recurrent feelings of estrangement were not due to our cultural differences in forms of politeness, manners of speech, attitudes towards time, or even differences in our aesthetic sensibilities (to me, at that time, Beethoven was just so much noise while I doubt if he even knew of the existence of Hindustani classical music which so moved me). The estrangement involved much deeper cultural layers of the self, such as fundamental ideas about the body, human relationships, family, marriage, male, and female which were an irreducible part of my subjectivity as, I suppose, they were a part of his. In other words, if during a session we sometimes suddenly became strangers to each other, it was because each of us found himself locked into a specific cultural unconscious, consisting of a more or less closed system of cultural representations that were not easily accessible to conscious awareness. Glimmers of these deeper cultural layers became visible, although I did not fully recognize them until many years after the analysis ended.

At first, I registered the role of culture in my analysis as a series of niggling feelings of discomfort whose source remained incomprehensible for many months. Indeed, many years were to pass before I began to comprehend the cultural landscape of the mind in more than a rudimentary fashion and make some sense of my experiences, both as an analysand and as an analyst, in cross-cultural therapeutic dyads (Kakar, 1982, 1987, 1989, 1994, 1997).

What could my analyst have done? Did he need to acquire knowledge of my culture, and if so, what kind of knowledge? Would an anthropological, historical, or philosophical grounding in Hindu culture have made him understand me better? Or was it a *psychoanalytical* knowledge of my culture that would have been more helpful? Psychoanalytical knowledge of a culture is not equivalent to its anthropological knowledge, although there may be some overlap between the two. Psychoanalytic knowledge is primarily the knowledge of the culture's *imagination*, of its fantasy as encoded in its symbolic products – its myths and folktales, its popular art, literature, and cinema.

Besides asking about the kind of knowledge, we also need to ask the question "Which culture?" Would a psychoanalytic knowledge of Hindu culture have been sufficient in my case? Yes, I am a Hindu, but also a Punjabi Khatri by birth. That is, my overarching Hindu culture has been mediated by my strong regional culture as a Punjabi and further by my Khatri caste. This Hindu Punjabi Khatri culture has been further modified by an agnostic father and a more traditional, believing mother, both of whom were also westernized to varying degrees. Is it not too much to expect any analyst to acquire this kind of prior cultural knowledge about his patients? On the other hand, is it okay for the analyst not to have *any* knowledge of his patient's cultural background? Or does the truth, as it often does, lie somewhere in the middle?

But now comes the surprise. My analyst was very good – sensitive, insightful, patient. And I discovered that as my analysis progressed, my feelings of estrangement that had given rise to all these questions became fewer and fewer. What was happening? Was the cultural part of my self becoming less salient as the analysis touched ever-deeper layers of the self, as many psychoanalysts have claimed?

Most analysts have followed George Deveraux's (1953) lead in maintaining that all those who seek help from a psychoanalyst have in common many fundamental and universal components in their personality structure. Together with the universality of the psychoanalytic method, these common factors sufficiently equip the analyst to understand and help his patient, irrespective of the patient's cultural background, a view reiterated by a panel of the American Psychoanalytic on the role of culture in psychoanalysis more than forty-five years ago (Jackson, 1968). There are certainly difficulties such as the ones enumerated by Ticho (1971) in treating patients of a different culture: a temporary impairment of the analyst's technical skills, empathy for the patient, diagnostic acumen, the stability of self and object representations, and the stirring up of counter-transference manifestations which may not be easily distinguishable from stereotypical reactions to the foreign culture. Generally, though, given the analyst's empathetic stance and the rules of analytic procedure, these difficulties are temporary and do not require a change in analytic technique. It is useful but not essential for the analyst to understand the patient's cultural heritage.

I believe that these conclusions on the role of culture in psychoanalytic therapy, which would seem to apply to my own experience, are superficially true but deeply mistaken. For what I did, and I believe most patients do, was to enthusiastically, if unconsciously, acculturate to the analyst's culture – in my case, both to his broader Western, north-European culture and to his particular Freudian psychoanalytic culture. The latter, we know, is informed by a vision of human experience that emphasizes man's individuality and his self-contained psyche. In the psychoanalytic vision, in Kenneth Kenniston's words (Adams, 1979), each of us lives in his own subjective world, pursuing pleasures and private fantasies, constructing a life and a fate which will vanish when our time is over. It emphasizes the desirability of reflective awareness of one's inner states, insistence that our psyches harbor deeper secrets than we care to confess, the existence of an objective reality that can be known, and an essential complexity and tragedy of life where many wishes are fated to remain unfulfilled. I was, then, moving from my own Hindu cultural heritage that sees life not as tragic but as a romantic quest that can extend over many births, with the goal and possibility of apprehending another, "higher" level of reality beyond the shared, verifiable, empirical reality of our world, our bodies, and our emotions.

Now, we know that every form of therapy is also an enculturation. As Fancher (1993) remarks:

> By the questions we ask, the things we empathize with, the themes we pick for our comment, the ways we conduct ourselves toward the patient, the language we use – by all these and a host of other ways, we communicate to the patient our notions [Freudian, Jungian, Kleinian, Lacanian etc.] of what is 'normal' and normative. Our interpretations [Freudian, Jungian, Kleinian, Lacanian etc.] of the origins of a patient's issues reveal in pure form our assumptions of what causes what, what is problematic about life, where the patient did not get what s/he needed, what should have been otherwise.
>
> *(pp. 89–90)*

As a patient in throes of transference love, I was exquisitely attuned to the cues to my analyst's values, beliefs, and vision of the fulfilled life, which even the most non-intrusive of analysts cannot help but scatter during the therapeutic process. I was quick to pick up the cues that unconsciously shaped my reactions and responses accordingly, with their overriding goal to please and be pleasing in the eyes of the beloved analyst. My intense need to be "understood" by the analyst, a need I shared with every patient, gave birth to an unconscious force that made me underplay those cultural parts of my self which I believed would be too foreign to the analyst's experience. In the transference love, what I sought was closeness to the analyst, including the sharing of his culturally shaped interests, attitudes, and beliefs. This intense need to be close and to be understood, paradoxically by removing parts of the self from the analytic arena of understanding, was epitomized by the fact that I soon started dreaming in German, the language of my analyst, something I have not done before or after my analysis.

This tendency to excise cultural part of the self is accelerated when the therapy is conducted in a language other than the mother tongue wherein much of one's native culture is encoded. One's mother tongue, the language of one's childhood, is intimately linked with emotionally colored sensory-motor experiences. Psychoanalysis in a language that is not the patient's own is often in danger of leading to "operational thinking," that is, verbal expressions lacking associational links with feelings, symbols, and memories (Basch-Kahre, 1984). However grammatically correct and rich in its vocabulary, the alien language suffers from emotional poverty, certainly as far as early memories are concerned.

The emotional poverty of language that is acquired much later has been dramatically demonstrated by an experiment in which subjects are asked the following question. A train is approaching at high speed. If you can push one individual on the track, stopping the train, it will save the lives of six others standing a little distance down the track. Will you push that individual in front of the train? Asked and answered in the mother tongue, most people show signs of an emotional dilemma and would not push the person to his death. The same question in the acquired language evokes much greater calculated rationality and the readiness to push one person in order to save the lives of six.

How should a psychotherapist, then, approach the issue of cultural difference of his client in his practice? The ideal situation would be that this difference exists only minimally, in the sense that the psychoanalytical therapist has obtained a psychoanalytic knowledge of the patient's culture through a long immersion in its daily life and its myths, its folklore and literature, its language and its music – an absorption not through the bones, as in case of his patient, but through the head – and the heart. Anything less than this maximalist position has the danger of the analyst succumbing to the lure of cultural stereotyping in dealing with the particularities of the patient's experience. In cross-cultural therapeutic dyads, little knowledge is indeed a dangerous thing, collapsing important differences, assuming sameness when only similarities exist. What the analyst needs is not a detailed knowledge of the patient's culture but a serious questioning and awareness of the assumptions underlying his own, i.e. the culture he was born into and the culture in which he has been professionally socialized as a psychoanalyst. In other words, what I am suggesting is that in absence of the possibility of obtaining a deep psychoanalytic knowledge of his patient's culture, the analyst needs to strive for a state of affairs where the patient's feelings of estrangement because of his cultural differences from the analyst are minimized, and the patient does not cut, or only minimally cuts, off the cultural part of the self from the therapeutic situation. This is possible only if the analyst can convey a cultural openness which comes from becoming aware of his culture's fundamental propositions about human nature, human experience, the fulfilled human life, and then to acknowledge their relativity by seeing them as cultural products, embedded in a particular place and time. He needs to become sensitive to the hidden existence of what Kohut (1979, p. 12) called "health and maturity moralities" of his particular analytical school. He needs to root out cultural judgments about what constitutes psychological maturity, gender-appropriate behaviors, "positive" or "negative" resolutions of developmental conflicts and complexes, that often appear in the garb of universally valid truths.

Given that ethnocentrism, the tendency to view alien cultures in terms of our own, and unresolved cultural chauvinism, are the patrimony of all human beings, including that of psychoanalysts, the acquisition of cultural openness is not an easy task. Cultural biases can lurk in the most unlikely places. For instance, to judge from the number of articles in psychoanalytic journals and books, psychoanalysis has traditionally accorded a high place to artistic creativity. To paint, sculpt, engage in literary and musical pursuits have not always and everywhere enjoyed the high prestige they do in modern Western societies. In other historical periods, many civilizations, including mine to this day, placed religious creativity at the top of their scale of desirable human endeavors. Psychoanalysts need to imagine that in such cultural settings, the following conclusion to a case report could be an example of a successful therapeutic outcome: "The patient's visions increased markedly in quantity and quality and the devotional mood took hold of her for longer and longer periods of time."

I would suggest that for optimal psychotherapy with patients from different cultures, what a psychoanalytical therapist needs is not an exhaustive knowledge of the patient's culture but a reflective openness to and interrogation of his own cultural origins. A therapist can evaluate his progress toward this openness by the increase in his feelings of curiosity and wonder in his counter-transference when the cultural parts of the patient's self find their voice in therapy, when the temptation to pathologize the cultural part of his patient's behavior decreases, when his own values no longer appear as normal and virtuous and when his wish to instruct the patient in these values diminishes markedly.

References

Adams, V. (1979). Freud's work thrives as theory, not therapy. *The New York Times*, 14 August.

Basch-Kahre, E. (1984). On difficulties arising in transference and countertransference when analyst and analysand have different socio-cultural backgrounds. *International Review of Psychoanalysis*, 11: 61–67.

Deveraux, G. (1953). Cultural factors in psychoanalytic therapy. *Journal of the American Psychoanalytic Association*, 1: 629–655.

Fancher, R.T. (1993). Psychoanalysis as culture. *Issues in Psychoanalytic Psychology*, 15(2): 81–93.

Jackson, S. (1968). Panel on aspects of culture in psychoanalytic theory and practice. *Journal of the American Psychoanalytic Association*, 16: 651–670.

Kakar, S. (1982). *Shamans, Mystics and Doctors*. New York: Knopf.

Kakar, S. (1987). Psychoanalysis and non-western cultures. *International Review of Psychoanalysis*, 12: 441–448.

Kakar, S. (1989). The maternal-feminine in Indian psychoanalysis. *International Review of Psychoanalysis*, 16(3): 355–362.

Kakar, S. (1994). Clinical work and cultural imagination. *Psychoanalytic Quarterly*, 64: 265–281.

Kakar, S. (1997). *Culture and Psyche*. New Delhi: Oxford University Press.

Kohut, H. (1979). The two analyses of Mr. Z. *International Journal of Psycho-Analysis*, 60: 12.

Ticho, G. (1971). Cultural aspects of transference and countertransference. *Bulletin of the Menninger Clinic*, 35(5): 313–326.

INDEX

For Product Safety Concerns and Information please contact our EU representative GPSR@taylorandfrancis.com
Taylor & Francis Verlag GmbH, Kaufingerstraße 24, 80331 München, Germany

www.ingramcontent.com/pod-product-compliance
Ingram Content Group UK Ltd.
Pitfield, Milton Keynes, MK11 3LW, UK
UKHW020205200926
475702UK00004B/630
9780367182458